NARCOLEPSY DIET COOKBOOK FOR BEGINNERS

Delicious Recipes and Nutritional Strategies for Managing Sleep Disorders and Boosting Daily Energy

Kingsley Klopp

To show our appreciation for your purchase, we're delighted to offer you these special bonuses as a heartfelt thank you

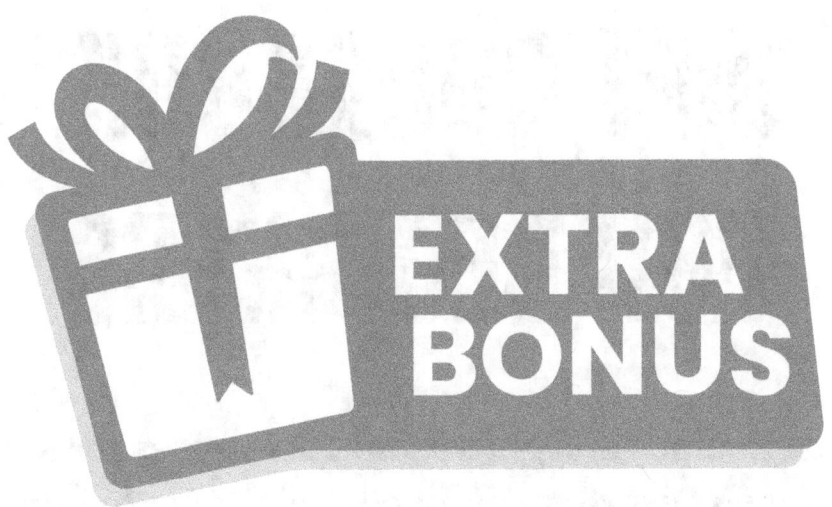

1. A Food Tracker Journal
2. Downloadable E-BOOK featuring full-color images of finished recipes

Copyright © 2024 All rights reserved.
No part of this book may be reproduced or transmitted in any form or by any means, electronic or mechanical, including photocopying, recording, or by any information storage and retrieval system, without written permission from the author. The scanning, uploading, and distribution of this book via the internet or via any other means without the permission of the author is illegal and punishable by law. The author has made every effort to ensure the accuracy of the information contained in this book. However, the author cannot be held responsible for any errors or omissions.

Table of Contents

Introduction...7

Part 1
Understanding Narcolepsy
- What is Narcolepsy?...9
- Symptoms and Diagnosis..11
- How Diet Affects Narcolepsy..13

Part 2
Key Nutrients for Managing Narcolepsy
- Protein..15
- Healthy Fats..17
- Fiber...19
- Vitamins and Minerals...21

Foods to Avoid..23

Breakfast Recipes
Spinach and Feta Omelette...25
Greek Yogurt Parfait with Nuts and Berries...............................26
Almond Butter Banana Smoothie...27
Turkey and Spinach Scramble..28
Protein Pancakes..29
Vegetable Stir-Fry with Tofu...30
Quinoa Porridge..31
Egg Muffins with Veggies and Cheese..32
Kale and Sweet Potato Hash..33
Low Carb Blueberry Muffins...34
Zucchini and Carrot Fritters...35
Overnight Oats with Flaxseed...36
Chicken Sausage Breakfast Burrito..37
Pumpkin Seed Granola..38

Soy and Linseed Porridge..39
Buckwheat Pancakes...40
Beetroot and Ginger Smoothie...41
Tuna Salad on Whole Wheat Toast..41
Asparagus and Mushroom Frittata..42
Muesli with Skim Milk..43
Protein-Packed Lentil Salad...43
 Sweet Potato and Black Bean Breakfast Bowl..44
Tempeh and Broccoli Sauté...45
Almond Flour Waffles...46
Oat Bran Muffin..47

Poultry Recipes
Grilled Chicken with Avocado Salsa...48
Turkey Lettuce Wraps..49
Chicken and Vegetable Stir-Fry...50
Baked Lemon Herb Chicken..51
Ground Turkey Stuffed Peppers..52
Spicy Chicken and Hummus Pita..53
Turkey Meatball Soup..54
Cajun Chicken Quinoa Bowl..55
Balsamic Glazed Chicken Breasts...56
Chicken Ratatouille..57
Mushroom and Spinach Stuffed Chicken...58
Chicken and Broccoli Alfredo..59
Curried Chicken Salad...60
Garlic and Herb Roasted Turkey Breast...61
Turkey and Sweet Potato Skillet...62
Buffalo Chicken Stuffed Zucchini Boats...63
Pesto Chicken Wraps...64
Herb-Roasted Chicken Thighs..65
Lemon Garlic Turkey Burgers...66
BBQ Turkey Meatloaf...67
Chicken Vegetable Soup..68
Asian Sesame Chicken Salad..69
Chicken and Spinach Stuffed Sweet Potatoes...70
Turkey and Quinoa Meatballs...71
Chicken and Lentil Stew..72

Fish and Seafood Recipes
Grilled Salmon with Lemon Dill Sauce...73
Shrimp and Avocado Salad..74

Baked Cod with Herb Crust...75
Tuna Nicoise Salad..76
Seafood Paella..77
Fish Tacos with Cabbage Slaw...78
 Grilled Mackerel with Orange Salad..79
Smoked Salmon and Cream Cheese Omelette..80
Scallop and Pea Risotto..81
Mediterranean Baked Trout..82
Pan-Seared Tilapia with Tomato Caper Sauce...83
Spicy Shrimp Stir-Fry...84
Salmon Quinoa Burgers..85
Fish Curry with Vegetables..86
Pistachio-Crusted Halibut..87
Oyster Mushroom and Shrimp Ramen...88
Thai Coconut Fish Soup...89
Sesame Seared Tuna..90
Garlic Butter Scallops..91
Grilled Shrimp and Pineapple Skewers..92
Squid Ink Pasta with Seafood..93
Lemon Pepper Haddock...94
Bouillabaisse...95
Seared Scallops with Mango Salsa..96
Anchovy and Broccoli Pasta..97

Vegetables
Roasted Cauliflower with Turmeric and Cumin..98
Kale and Quinoa Salad with Lemon Vinaigrette...99
Stuffed Bell Peppers with Brown Rice and Vegetables...............................100
Spicy Roasted Sweet Potatoes...101
Zucchini Noodles with Pesto and Cherry Tomatoes...................................102
Grilled Eggplant with Tahini Sauce..103
Beetroot and Feta Salad..104
Broccoli and Almond Stir-Fry...105
Spinach and Mushroom Quiche...106
Cabbage Slaw with Apple Cider Vinegar Dressing.....................................107
 Asparagus and Feta Omelette...108
Butternut Squash Risotto..109
Vegetable Paella with Saffron..110
Stir-Fried Bok Choy with Garlic and Soy Sauce..111
Cucumber and Dill Salad with Yogurt Dressing..112
Tomato Gazpacho..113
Mushroom and Barley Soup...114

Curried Lentils with Spinach and Carrots..115
Sweet Potato and Chickpea Curry...116
Roasted Parsnips and Carrots with Honey Glaze..117
Creamy Avocado Spinach Pasta..118
Vegan Cauliflower Tacos..119
Green Bean Almondine..120
Stuffed Portobello Mushrooms with Quinoa...121
Leek and Potato Gratin..122

10-WEEK MEAL PLAN..**123**

Important Note

Thank you for picking up the **Narcolepsy Diet Cookbook**. We're thrilled to be part of your journey towards better health and more vibrant living. As you dive into these pages filled with delicious and nutritious recipes, we want to share an important note with you.

Each of us is unique, and our bodies respond differently to various foods. While the recipes in this book are crafted to support those living with narcolepsy, it's essential to remember that individual dietary needs may vary. What works wonderfully for one person may not be as effective for another. Therefore, we encourage you to adjust these recipes to suit your personal preferences and nutritional requirements. We highly recommend consulting with your healthcare provider or a registered dietitian before making significant changes to your diet, especially if you have specific health concerns or dietary restrictions. They can offer personalized guidance and ensure that your dietary adjustments align with your overall health plan.

Additionally, please note that the nutritional information provided in this cookbook is approximate. Variations in ingredients, preparation methods, and serving sizes can affect the nutritional content of each dish. We've done our best to provide accurate estimates, but they should be used as a general guide rather than an exact measure.

Furthermore, If our cookbook has brought joy to your kitchen and table, we'd be thrilled to hear about your experiences in an Amazon review. On the flip side, if you stumble upon any hiccups while exploring our recipes, don't hesitate to get in touch at kloppkingsley@gmail.com. We're here to support your cooking journey every step of the way.

Our goal is to empower you with knowledge and inspire you to create meals that enhance your wellbeing. We hope you find joy in experimenting with these recipes and discovering what best supports your health and lifestyle.

Introduction.

Welcome to the **Narcolepsy Diet Cookbook for Beginners**. If you're reading this, chances are you or someone you love is living with narcolepsy. You're likely familiar with the unpredictable sleepiness, the overwhelming fatigue, and the constant struggle to maintain a sense of normalcy. You're not alone. Narcolepsy affects millions of people worldwide, and while medication and lifestyle changes play a crucial role in managing this condition, there's an often-overlooked hero in this journey: food.

Yes, you read that right. The food you eat can have a significant impact on your narcolepsy symptoms. Imagine waking up feeling more rested, having stable energy throughout the day, and experiencing fewer unexpected bouts of sleepiness. This might sound like a dream, but with the right diet, it can become your reality.

This cookbook is your companion in discovering how the right foods can fuel your body, stabilize your energy levels, and help you regain control over your daily life. It's not just about eating healthy; it's about eating smart. Each recipe in this book is crafted with ingredients known to support brain health, promote steady energy, and avoid common dietary pitfalls that can exacerbate narcolepsy symptoms. Why a cookbook, you ask? Because food is more than just sustenance. It's comfort, it's culture, it's connection. And when you're managing a condition like narcolepsy, food can also be a powerful tool for healing and wellness. This cookbook isn't just about providing recipes; it's about empowering you with the knowledge and tools you need to make food choices that support your health and wellbeing. Narcolepsy can be an isolating condition, but it doesn't have to be. Through these pages, you'll find a community of individuals who have navigated similar challenges and discovered the transformative power of diet. You'll read about the science behind certain foods and their effects on narcolepsy, and you'll gain practical tips for meal planning, grocery shopping, and dining out.

Let's start with the basics. Narcolepsy is a chronic sleep disorder characterized by overwhelming daytime drowsiness and sudden attacks of sleep. It can profoundly affect your quality of life, making it difficult to perform daily activities, maintain employment, and enjoy social interactions. While medications can help manage symptoms, they often come with side effects and may not be fully effective for everyone. This is where diet comes into play. Emerging research suggests that certain dietary patterns can influence sleep and energy levels. For example, diets high in refined sugars and carbohydrates can lead to spikes and crashes in blood sugar, which may exacerbate narcolepsy symptoms. On the other hand, a diet rich in lean proteins, healthy fats, fiber, and essential vitamins and minerals can promote steady energy levels and improve overall wellbeing.

In this cookbook, you'll find a variety of recipes tailored to support your journey with narcolepsy. From energizing breakfasts that will help you kickstart your day, to balanced lunches that prevent afternoon slumps, and hearty dinners that promote restful sleep, each recipe is designed with your unique needs in mind. You'll also discover snacks that keep your energy stable and drinks that hydrate without causing drowsiness. We understand that starting a new diet can feel overwhelming, especially when dealing with a chronic condition. That's why this book is designed to be as user-friendly as possible. Each recipe includes clear instructions, nutritional information, and practical tips for making meal prep easier. Whether you're a seasoned cook or a kitchen novice, you'll find recipes that fit your skill level and lifestyle.

So, are you ready to transform your relationship with food and take a proactive step in managing your narcolepsy? Let's embark on this journey together. Grab your apron, fire up the stove, and let's create meals that nourish your body, support your health, and bring joy back to your table. Welcome to the **Narcolepsy Diet Cookbook for Beginners** – your guide to eating well and living better.

Part 1

Understanding Narcolepsy

What is Narcolepsy?

Narcolepsy is a complex and often misunderstood neurological disorder that profoundly affects the lives of those who live with it. Imagine feeling a constant, overwhelming sense of tiredness, regardless of how much rest you've had. This is the daily reality for people with narcolepsy. It's not just about feeling sleepy; it's about the body and brain being unable to regulate sleep-wake cycles properly, leading to a cascade of challenges that affect every aspect of life. At its core, narcolepsy disrupts the natural boundaries between sleep and wakefulness. In a healthy individual, these boundaries are distinct, with sleep occurring primarily at night and wakefulness dominating the day. However, for those with narcolepsy, these boundaries are blurred. They might fall asleep suddenly during the day, even in the middle of activities like eating, talking, or driving, a phenomenon known as "*sleep attacks.*" These sleep attacks can be incredibly dangerous and are one of the most striking and disruptive aspects of the disorder. But narcolepsy is much more than just these sleep attacks. It is a disorder that touches every corner of a person's life. The constant fatigue and sudden bouts of sleepiness can make it incredibly challenging to maintain a job, keep up with school, or even enjoy social activities. The unpredictability of the condition can lead to feelings of embarrassment, isolation, and frustration. It's not uncommon for people with narcolepsy to feel misunderstood by those around them, who might mistake their symptoms for laziness or lack of motivation.

Narcolepsy is generally categorized into two types: *Type 1*, which includes cataplexy (a sudden loss of muscle tone triggered by strong emotions), and *Type 2*, which does not. Cataplexy can be particularly distressing, as it can cause individuals to collapse suddenly, potentially injuring themselves. This symptom, unique to Type 1 narcolepsy, often brings a great deal of emotional turmoil, as people may fear experiencing cataplexy in public or during important moments. One of the most heart-wrenching aspects of narcolepsy is its impact on mental health. The constant struggle to stay awake and the embarrassment of sleep attacks can lead to anxiety and depression. The lack of understanding and support from others can exacerbate these feelings, making individuals with narcolepsy feel even more isolated. It's not just a battle against sleepiness; it's a battle for normalcy, acceptance, and understanding.

The cause of narcolepsy is still not entirely understood, but it is believed to involve a combination of genetic and environmental factors. In many cases, it is linked to a deficiency of hypocretin (also known as orexin), a neurotransmitter in the brain that plays a crucial role in regulating wakefulness and REM (rapid eye movement) sleep. This deficiency can be caused by an autoimmune response, where the body's immune system mistakenly attacks and destroys hypocretin-producing cells. Living with narcolepsy requires significant adjustments and a great deal of resilience. Individuals must learn to manage their condition through lifestyle changes, medications, and often, the support of a healthcare team. This might include establishing a strict sleep schedule, taking scheduled naps during the day, and avoiding activities that could be dangerous during a sleep attack.

Despite these challenges, many people with narcolepsy find ways to lead fulfilling lives. They become adept at planning and managing their symptoms, seeking out supportive communities, and advocating for greater awareness and understanding of their condition. Their journey is one of perseverance and determination, continually adapting to the unpredictable nature of their disorder. For those who have narcolepsy, understanding their condition is the first step toward reclaiming control over their lives. It's about acknowledging the struggle, embracing the support of loved ones, and finding the strength within themselves to navigate the challenges that lie ahead. Narcolepsy may be a lifelong condition, but with the right tools and support, individuals can find ways to thrive and live their lives to the fullest.

Symptoms and Diagnosis of Narcolepsy

Symptoms of Narcolepsy

1. Excessive Daytime Sleepiness (EDS):
   - The hallmark symptom of narcolepsy is excessive daytime sleepiness. Individuals with narcolepsy experience an overwhelming urge to sleep during the day, regardless of how much rest they had the night before. This sleepiness can strike at any time, leading to "sleep attacks" where a person may fall asleep suddenly and without warning, often during activities like talking, eating, or driving. This can severely affect daily functioning and quality of life.
2. Cataplexy:
   - Cataplexy is a sudden, brief loss of muscle tone triggered by strong emotions such as laughter, anger, or surprise. This can cause a range of effects, from mild weakness (such as a slackening of the jaw) to complete collapse. Cataplexy is unique to Type 1 narcolepsy and can be distressing and dangerous, especially if it occurs in situations where falling could lead to injury.
3. Sleep Paralysis:
   - Sleep paralysis involves a temporary inability to move or speak while falling asleep or waking up. During these episodes, which typically last a few seconds to a few minutes, individuals are fully conscious but unable to control their muscles. This can be a frightening experience, especially when accompanied by hallucinations.
4. Hypnagogic and Hypnopompic Hallucinations:
   - These vivid and often frightening hallucinations occur while falling asleep (hypnagogic) or waking up (hypnopompic). They can involve any of the senses, such as seeing shadowy figures, hearing voices, or feeling a presence in the room. These hallucinations are typically associated with the transition between wakefulness and sleep.
5. Disrupted Nighttime Sleep:
   - Despite excessive daytime sleepiness, many individuals with narcolepsy also experience fragmented nighttime sleep, waking up multiple times during the night. This can lead to difficulty maintaining consistent and restorative sleep, exacerbating daytime symptoms.
6. Automatic Behaviors:
   - During periods of extreme sleepiness, individuals with narcolepsy may perform routine tasks without full awareness or memory of doing so. These automatic behaviors can include actions like eating, writing, or driving, and can pose significant risks, especially in situations requiring full attention.

Diagnosis of Narcolepsy

Diagnosing narcolepsy involves a comprehensive evaluation by a sleep specialist, as the symptoms can overlap with other sleep disorders and medical conditions. The diagnostic process typically includes:

1. Medical History and Symptom Assessment:
   - The first step in diagnosing narcolepsy is a thorough medical history and detailed description of symptoms. The doctor will ask about the frequency, duration, and severity of sleepiness and other related symptoms. It's essential to discuss any family history of sleep disorders and other medical conditions that might be contributing to the symptoms.

2. Sleep Diary and Questionnaires:
   - Patients may be asked to keep a sleep diary for one to two weeks, recording sleep patterns, naps, and any occurrences of cataplexy, sleep paralysis, or hallucinations. Additionally, standardized questionnaires like the Epworth Sleepiness Scale may be used to assess the level of daytime sleepiness.

3. Polysomnography (PSG):
   - Polysomnography is an overnight sleep study conducted in a sleep laboratory. It monitors various physiological parameters, including brain waves, heart rate, breathing patterns, and eye movements, to evaluate sleep architecture and identify any abnormalities. PSG helps rule out other sleep disorders, such as sleep apnea, that could be causing excessive daytime sleepiness.

4. Multiple Sleep Latency Test (MSLT):
   - The MSLT is a daytime nap study usually conducted the day after polysomnography. During the MSLT, the patient is given several opportunities to nap at two-hour intervals throughout the day. The test measures how quickly the patient falls asleep and how quickly they enter rapid eye movement (REM) sleep. Short sleep latency (falling asleep in less than eight minutes) and early onset of REM sleep in at least two of the five naps strongly suggest narcolepsy.

5. Hypocretin Level Measurement:
   - In some cases, especially when cataplexy is present, cerebrospinal fluid (CSF) analysis may be performed to measure the levels of hypocretin-1 (also known as orexin-A). Low levels of this neurotransmitter, which regulates wakefulness, are indicative of narcolepsy Type 1. This test involves a lumbar puncture to collect the CSF sample.

6. Genetic Testing:
   - Genetic testing may be conducted to identify the presence of specific human leukocyte antigen (HLA) subtypes, such as HLA-DQB1*06:02, which are associated with an increased risk of narcolepsy. However, genetic testing alone is not sufficient for diagnosis as not all individuals with these markers develop narcolepsy.

How Diet Affects Narcolepsy

Living with narcolepsy can be a relentless battle, where the line between wakefulness and sleep is a constant blur. Yet, in this challenging journey, the role of diet offers a beacon of hope. The food we consume has a profound impact on our health and well-being, and for those with narcolepsy, making mindful dietary choices can be transformative. Diet is more than just fuel; it's a source of sustenance, comfort, and sometimes even joy. For people with narcolepsy, it becomes a vital part of managing the condition. Imagine waking up feeling perpetually exhausted, your body betraying you with sudden bouts of sleepiness. Now, envision a life where strategic dietary choices help to stabilize your energy levels, enhance your alertness, and mitigate the overwhelming fatigue. This is the potential power of a narcolepsy-friendly diet.

Energy Regulation

One of the most significant ways diet affects narcolepsy is through energy regulation. Foods rich in complex carbohydrates, proteins, and healthy fats provide a steady release of energy throughout the day, helping to combat the sudden and intense waves of sleepiness that characterize narcolepsy. Complex carbohydrates, found in whole grains, legumes, and vegetables, are digested slowly, providing a gradual and sustained energy release. This can help to prevent the mid-morning or afternoon energy crashes that are so debilitating for those with narcolepsy. Proteins, found in lean meats, eggs, dairy, nuts, and seeds, are crucial for maintaining muscle health and energy levels. They also play a role in neurotransmitter production, which is essential for brain function and alertness. Healthy fats, such as those found in avocados, olive oil, and fatty fish, support brain health and can help to maintain energy levels. Together, these nutrients form the backbone of a balanced diet that can help manage narcolepsy symptoms.

Blood Sugar Stability

Blood sugar fluctuations can have a significant impact on energy levels and alertness. For individuals with narcolepsy, maintaining stable blood sugar levels is crucial. Spikes and crashes in blood sugar can exacerbate feelings of fatigue and sleepiness. Consuming meals and snacks that include a balance of carbohydrates, proteins, and fats can help to keep blood sugar levels steady. For example, pairing an apple with a handful of almonds provides a combination of carbs, protein, and healthy fats that will help sustain energy levels longer than a sugary snack alone.

Avoiding refined sugars and processed foods is particularly important. These foods can cause rapid spikes in blood sugar, followed by sharp declines, leading to increased fatigue and sleepiness. Instead, opting for whole, unprocessed foods that are high in fiber can help to maintain more consistent blood sugar levels.

Brain Health and Function

Diet also plays a critical role in brain health and function. Nutrients like omega-3 fatty acids, antioxidants, and vitamins B6 and B12 are essential for maintaining cognitive function and mental clarity. Omega-3 fatty acids, found in fish, flaxseeds, and walnuts, are known to support brain health and may help reduce inflammation. Antioxidants, found in fruits and vegetables, protect the brain from oxidative stress and damage. B vitamins are essential for energy production and brain function. For someone with narcolepsy, supporting brain health is paramount. Cognitive symptoms such as brain fog and difficulty concentrating can be as challenging as the sleepiness itself. A diet rich in brain-boosting nutrients can help to alleviate some of these cognitive symptoms, improving overall quality of life.

Weight Management

Weight management is another critical aspect of managing narcolepsy. Excess weight can exacerbate sleep problems and increase the risk of conditions like sleep apnea, which can further disrupt sleep quality. Eating a balanced diet and maintaining a healthy weight can help to improve sleep quality and reduce the severity of narcolepsy symptoms.

For those with narcolepsy, who may struggle with fatigue and find it challenging to stay active, managing weight through diet becomes even more important. Choosing nutrient-dense foods that provide the necessary vitamins and minerals without excess calories can help to support overall health and well-being.

Emotional and Mental Well-being

Finally, it's important to acknowledge the emotional and mental well-being that comes with a healthy diet. Living with narcolepsy can be incredibly isolating and frustrating. The unpredictability of symptoms can lead to feelings of anxiety, depression, and low self-esteem. By taking control of one's diet, individuals with narcolepsy can gain a sense of empowerment and hope. Preparing and enjoying nourishing meals can be a form of self-care, a way to show oneself love and compassion. It can also be an opportunity to connect with others, to share meals and experiences, and to find joy in the simple act of eating well.

Hence, while diet alone cannot cure narcolepsy, it is a powerful tool in managing its symptoms. By making mindful dietary choices, individuals with narcolepsy can improve their energy levels, stabilize blood sugar, support brain health, manage weight, and enhance their overall quality of life. It's a journey of small, daily choices that collectively make a significant impact, bringing light and hope to those navigating the challenges of narcolepsy.

Part 2

Key Nutrients for Managing Narcolepsy

Protein

Protein, one of the three macronutrients essential for human health, plays a crucial role in managing narcolepsy. For individuals living with this chronic neurological disorder, the right dietary choices can make a significant difference in their daily functioning and overall quality of life. Protein, in particular, offers a range of benefits that can help mitigate some of the symptoms of narcolepsy, providing a steady source of energy, supporting neurotransmitter function, and aiding in muscle maintenance and repair.

Steady Energy Supply

One of the most challenging aspects of narcolepsy is the overwhelming and unpredictable daytime sleepiness. Protein-rich foods can help provide a more sustained energy supply compared to simple carbohydrates, which can cause quick spikes and subsequent crashes in blood sugar levels. When proteins are broken down in the body, they provide a slow and steady release of energy, helping to maintain alertness and reduce the likelihood of sudden sleep attacks. For example, starting the day with a breakfast high in protein, such as eggs, Greek yogurt, or a protein smoothie, can help individuals feel more awake and alert throughout the morning. Incorporating protein into every meal and snack ensures a continuous energy supply, making it easier to manage the excessive daytime sleepiness that characterizes narcolepsy.

Neurotransmitter Function

Proteins are composed of amino acids, which are the building blocks of neurotransmitters – the chemicals that transmit signals in the brain. For those with narcolepsy, maintaining healthy neurotransmitter levels is crucial for managing sleep-wake cycles and cognitive function. Key neurotransmitters such as serotonin, dopamine, and norepinephrine are synthesized from amino acids found in protein-rich foods. For instance, tryptophan, an amino acid found in turkey, chicken, and dairy products, is a precursor to serotonin, which helps regulate mood and sleep. Tyrosine, found in eggs, dairy, and meat, is a precursor to dopamine and norepinephrine, which play roles in alertness and concentration. Ensuring a sufficient intake of these amino acids through a protein-rich diet can support the brain's ability to regulate sleep and maintain cognitive functions, such as memory and focus, which are often impaired in narcolepsy.

Muscle Maintenance and Repair

Narcolepsy can lead to a more sedentary lifestyle due to the constant fatigue and sudden sleep episodes. This sedentary behavior can result in muscle weakness and a decline in physical fitness. Protein is vital for muscle maintenance and repair, helping to counteract the effects of inactivity.

Including adequate protein in the diet can help individuals maintain muscle mass and strength, even if their activity levels are lower than desired. Lean meats, fish, beans, legumes, and plant-based proteins like tofu and tempeh are excellent sources of high-quality protein that support muscle health. Engaging in light to moderate physical activity, combined with a protein-rich diet, can help improve overall physical well-being and combat the lethargy associated with narcolepsy.

Satiety and Weight Management

Weight management is another critical aspect of managing narcolepsy. Excess weight can exacerbate sleep issues and increase the risk of conditions like sleep apnea, which can further disrupt sleep quality. Protein-rich foods are known for their ability to promote feelings of fullness and satiety, which can help control appetite and prevent overeating. High-protein foods like lean meats, fish, eggs, and legumes can help regulate hunger hormones and reduce cravings for unhealthy snacks, which are often high in sugars and refined carbohydrates. By helping to maintain a healthy weight, a protein-rich diet can indirectly contribute to better sleep quality and overall health, making it easier to manage the symptoms of narcolepsy.

Healthy Fats

Living with narcolepsy presents a unique set of challenges, particularly when it comes to maintaining energy levels and cognitive function. While many people focus on carbohydrates and proteins, healthy fats are equally crucial for managing this chronic condition. These fats not only provide a long-lasting energy source but also support brain health, help stabilize mood, and aid in the absorption of essential vitamins. Let's delve into how incorporating healthy fats into your diet can significantly impact the management of narcolepsy.

Sustained Energy Release

One of the primary benefits of healthy fats is their ability to provide a slow and steady source of energy. Unlike carbohydrates, which can cause quick spikes and drops in blood sugar levels, fats are metabolized more slowly, offering a sustained release of energy. For individuals with narcolepsy, this can be particularly beneficial in maintaining alertness and reducing the frequency and severity of daytime sleepiness. Including sources of healthy fats in meals and snacks can help ensure a consistent energy supply throughout the day. For instance, avocados, nuts, seeds, and fatty fish like salmon or mackerel are excellent choices that can be easily incorporated into various meals. Starting the day with a breakfast that includes healthy fats, such as avocado toast or a smoothie with nut butter, can help stabilize energy levels from the get-go.

Brain Health and Cognitive Function

Healthy fats, particularly omega-3 fatty acids, play a crucial role in brain health. These essential fats are integral components of cell membranes in the brain and are involved in numerous cognitive functions, including memory and mood regulation. Omega-3 fatty acids, found in high concentrations in fatty fish, flaxseeds, chia seeds, and walnuts, have been shown to support cognitive function and may help alleviate some of the cognitive symptoms associated with narcolepsy, such as brain fog and difficulty concentrating. Regular consumption of omega-3-rich foods can help support overall brain health, potentially improving mental clarity and focus. This is especially important for individuals with narcolepsy, as maintaining cognitive function can be challenging due to the disorder's impact on sleep and wakefulness cycles.

Mood Stabilization

Living with narcolepsy often comes with emotional challenges. The frustration and isolation that can accompany this condition may lead to anxiety and depression. Healthy fats, particularly omega-3 fatty acids, have been shown to have a positive effect on mood and emotional well-being. These fats help regulate the production of neurotransmitters like serotonin and dopamine, which are crucial for mood stabilization.

Incorporating omega-3-rich foods into your diet can support mental health, helping to stabilize mood and reduce the risk of depression. This can make it easier to cope with the emotional aspects of narcolepsy, fostering a more positive outlook and improving overall quality of life.

Absorption of Essential Vitamins
Healthy fats are essential for the absorption of fat-soluble vitamins such as vitamins A, D, E, and K. These vitamins play vital roles in various bodily functions, including immune function, bone health, and antioxidant protection. For individuals with narcolepsy, ensuring adequate intake and absorption of these vitamins is crucial for maintaining overall health and supporting the body's resilience.

For example, pairing a salad with a dressing made from olive oil or adding avocado to a meal can enhance the absorption of these essential vitamins from the vegetables. This not only boosts nutrient intake but also supports overall health and well-being.

Anti-inflammatory Properties
Chronic inflammation is linked to numerous health issues, including cognitive decline and mood disorders. Healthy fats, particularly those found in fish oil and certain plant oils, have anti-inflammatory properties that can help reduce inflammation in the body. This is particularly beneficial for individuals with narcolepsy, as managing inflammation can help improve overall health and potentially reduce some of the secondary symptoms associated with the condition.

Including anti-inflammatory foods in your diet, such as fatty fish, flaxseeds, and walnuts, can help mitigate inflammation, supporting overall health and well-being.

Fiber

Living with narcolepsy is a daily struggle against overwhelming fatigue and sudden sleep attacks. While medication and lifestyle changes are often the primary treatments, diet also plays a crucial role in managing this condition. Among the essential nutrients, fiber stands out for its numerous benefits, including stabilizing energy levels, supporting digestive health, and helping maintain a healthy weight. Here's a detailed look at how fiber can be a powerful ally for those managing narcolepsy.

Stabilizing Energy Levels

One of the most challenging aspects of narcolepsy is the constant battle with excessive daytime sleepiness. This can be exacerbated by fluctuations in blood sugar levels, which lead to rapid energy peaks and crashes. Foods high in fiber, such as whole grains, legumes, fruits, and vegetables, are digested more slowly than simple carbohydrates. This slow digestion helps to maintain steady blood sugar levels, providing a more sustained and stable source of energy throughout the day.

For example, starting your day with a high-fiber breakfast, such as oatmeal topped with berries and nuts, can help you avoid the mid-morning energy slump. Similarly, incorporating fiber-rich snacks like apple slices with almond butter or a handful of mixed nuts can keep energy levels stable between meals. This stability is crucial for those with narcolepsy, helping to mitigate sudden bouts of sleepiness and maintain alertness.

Supporting Digestive Health

Fiber is essential for a healthy digestive system, which in turn can affect overall well-being and energy levels. There are two types of fiber: soluble and insoluble. Soluble fiber, found in foods like oats, beans, and apples, dissolves in water to form a gel-like substance, which helps to lower blood cholesterol and glucose levels. Insoluble fiber, found in whole grains, nuts, and vegetables, adds bulk to stool and helps food pass more quickly through the stomach and intestines. A healthy digestive system ensures that the body efficiently absorbs nutrients from food, which is particularly important for individuals with narcolepsy. Poor digestion can lead to nutrient deficiencies and exacerbate feelings of fatigue. By including a variety of fiber-rich foods in your diet, you can promote regular bowel movements, reduce the risk of constipation, and enhance overall digestive health.

Weight Management

Maintaining a healthy weight is important for everyone, but it is especially critical for those with narcolepsy. Excess weight can increase the risk of sleep apnea and other sleep disorders, further complicating sleep patterns and exacerbating symptoms. High-fiber foods are typically lower in calories and more filling than low-fiber options, which can help with weight management by reducing overall calorie intake.

Fiber-rich foods take longer to chew and digest, which can increase feelings of fullness and reduce hunger. This can prevent overeating and help maintain a healthy weight. For example, a diet that includes plenty of vegetables, fruits, whole grains, and legumes can help control appetite and support weight management efforts, making it easier to manage narcolepsy symptoms.

Blood Sugar Control

As mentioned earlier, fiber helps to regulate blood sugar levels, which is crucial for individuals with narcolepsy. Rapid spikes and drops in blood sugar can lead to sudden fatigue and exacerbate daytime sleepiness. Soluble fiber, in particular, slows the absorption of sugar into the bloodstream, helping to prevent these rapid changes. Including fiber-rich foods in your diet can help maintain consistent blood sugar levels. For instance, choosing whole fruits over fruit juices, whole grains over refined grains, and legumes over processed foods can make a significant difference. By keeping blood sugar levels stable, you can reduce the likelihood of energy crashes and improve overall alertness.

Gut Health and Microbiome

Recent research has highlighted the importance of gut health and its connection to overall well-being, including mental health and sleep. Fiber plays a crucial role in maintaining a healthy gut microbiome, the community of bacteria and other microorganisms living in the digestive tract. These microbes ferment fiber, producing short-chain fatty acids that have numerous health benefits, including anti-inflammatory effects and improved immune function. A healthy gut microbiome can influence the production of neurotransmitters and hormones that regulate sleep and mood. For individuals with narcolepsy, maintaining a healthy gut through a fiber-rich diet can support better sleep quality and overall health. Foods like chicory root, garlic, onions, and bananas are excellent sources of prebiotic fiber that nourish beneficial gut bacteria.

Vitamins and Minerals

Vitamin B12 and Folate (Vitamin B9)
Vitamin B12 and folate are vital for the production of red blood cells and the maintenance of the nervous system. They are involved in the synthesis of DNA and RNA and are essential for proper brain function. Deficiencies in these vitamins can lead to fatigue, weakness, and neurological issues, which can exacerbate the symptoms of narcolepsy.
- Sources: Vitamin B12 is primarily found in animal products such as meat, fish, poultry, eggs, and dairy. For those following a vegetarian or vegan diet, fortified foods and supplements may be necessary. Folate is abundant in leafy green vegetables, legumes, nuts, and seeds.

Vitamin D
Vitamin D plays a crucial role in maintaining bone health, immune function, and mood regulation. There is emerging evidence suggesting that vitamin D may influence sleep patterns and quality. A deficiency in vitamin D has been linked to increased daytime sleepiness, which can worsen narcolepsy symptoms.
- Sources: The body produces vitamin D when exposed to sunlight. It can also be obtained from foods such as fatty fish (salmon, mackerel), fortified dairy products, and egg yolks. Supplements may be necessary, especially for individuals with limited sun exposure.

Magnesium
Magnesium is involved in over 300 biochemical reactions in the body, including those that regulate muscle and nerve function, blood glucose control, and energy production. It also plays a role in sleep regulation and can help improve sleep quality, which is vital for individuals with narcolepsy.
- Sources: Magnesium-rich foods include leafy green vegetables, nuts, seeds, whole grains, and legumes. Incorporating these foods into daily meals can help ensure adequate magnesium intake.

Iron
Iron is essential for the production of hemoglobin, which carries oxygen in the blood. Low iron levels can lead to anemia, characterized by fatigue and weakness. Ensuring adequate iron intake can help maintain energy levels and reduce feelings of exhaustion in individuals with narcolepsy.
- Sources: Iron is found in red meat, poultry, fish, legumes, and fortified cereals. Plant-based sources of iron should be consumed with vitamin C-rich foods (like citrus fruits) to enhance absorption.

Calcium
Calcium is crucial for bone health and plays a role in muscle function, nerve signaling, and blood clotting. Adequate calcium intake supports overall health and well-being, which is essential for managing narcolepsy.
- Sources: Dairy products (milk, cheese, yogurt), leafy green vegetables, and fortified plant-based milks are excellent sources of calcium.

Zinc
Zinc supports immune function, wound healing, DNA synthesis, and cell division. It also plays a role in maintaining a healthy nervous system and can contribute to overall energy levels.
- Sources: Zinc is found in meat, shellfish, dairy products, nuts, seeds, and whole grains. Including a variety of these foods in the diet can help ensure adequate zinc intake.

Omega-3 Fatty Acids
Although not vitamins or minerals, omega-3 fatty acids are essential fats that support brain health and function. They have anti-inflammatory properties and can help improve mood and cognitive function, which are often impacted in individuals with narcolepsy.
- Sources: Omega-3 fatty acids are found in fatty fish (salmon, mackerel, sardines), flaxseeds, chia seeds, and walnuts. Incorporating these foods into the diet can provide numerous health benefits.

Foods to Avoid

Sugary Foods and Beverages
Why to Avoid: Sugary foods and beverages cause rapid spikes in blood sugar levels, followed by sharp declines. These fluctuations can lead to sudden bursts of energy followed by intense fatigue, which can be particularly problematic for individuals with narcolepsy. The temporary high energy might seem beneficial, but the subsequent crash can exacerbate daytime sleepiness and make it harder to stay awake and alert.
Examples to Avoid:
- Soda and sugary drinks
- Candy and sweets
- Pastries and baked goods made with refined sugars
- Sweetened cereals
- Ice cream and sugary desserts

Caffeine
Why to Avoid: While caffeine is often used to combat sleepiness, it can be a double-edged sword for people with narcolepsy. In moderate amounts, it might help improve alertness, but excessive caffeine consumption can lead to poor nighttime sleep quality. Over time, reliance on caffeine can create a cycle of dependence, where disrupted night sleep leads to increased daytime caffeine consumption, further disturbing sleep patterns.
Examples to Avoid:
- Coffee (especially in large quantities or close to bedtime)
- Energy drinks
- Certain teas (like black and green tea)
- Caffeinated sodas
- Chocolate and chocolate-flavored products

Processed Foods and Fast Food
Why to Avoid: Processed foods and fast food are often high in unhealthy fats, sugars, and sodium. These foods can cause inflammation, digestive issues, and contribute to poor overall health. Additionally, they are often low in essential nutrients, which can lead to nutrient deficiencies that exacerbate narcolepsy symptoms. The high levels of unhealthy fats and sugars can also contribute to weight gain, which can worsen sleep apnea and other sleep-related issues.
Examples to Avoid:
- Fast food (burgers, fries, fried chicken)
- Processed snacks (chips, crackers, instant noodles)
- Packaged baked goods (cookies, muffins, donuts)
- Frozen meals and pizza
- Sugary breakfast cereals

Alcohol

Why to Avoid: Alcohol can significantly disrupt sleep architecture by altering the natural sleep cycle. Although it might help induce sleep initially, it leads to fragmented sleep and reduces the amount of restorative REM sleep. For individuals with narcolepsy, maintaining a consistent and high-quality sleep pattern is crucial, and alcohol can severely interfere with this.

Examples to Avoid:
- Beer, Wine
- Spirits (whiskey, vodka, rum)
- Cocktails and mixed drinks

High-Glycemic Index Foods

Why to Avoid: High-glycemic index (GI) foods cause rapid increases in blood sugar levels, similar to sugary foods. These spikes can lead to energy crashes, worsening daytime sleepiness and making it difficult to manage narcolepsy symptoms. Foods with a high GI can also contribute to weight gain and increase the risk of developing insulin resistance and diabetes.

Examples to Avoid:
- White bread and refined flour products
- White rice
- Potatoes (especially mashed or fried)
- Instant oatmeal
- Certain breakfast cereals

Heavy, Fatty Foods

Why to Avoid: Heavy, fatty foods can be difficult to digest and may lead to feelings of sluggishness and lethargy. They can also cause digestive discomfort and disrupt sleep patterns, making it harder to achieve restful sleep. For those with narcolepsy, maintaining a diet that promotes steady energy levels and good digestion is essential.

Examples to Avoid:
- Fatty cuts of meat (like bacon, sausage, and certain beef cuts)
- Deep-fried foods (like fried chicken, fish, and chips)
- Full-fat dairy products (like cream, butter, and high-fat cheese)
- Rich, creamy sauces and gravies

Artificial Additives and Preservatives

Why to Avoid: Artificial additives and preservatives found in many processed foods can cause a range of adverse health effects, including allergic reactions, digestive issues, and inflammation. These additives can also disrupt normal bodily functions and exacerbate symptoms of narcolepsy by impacting overall health and well-being.

Examples to Avoid:
- Artificial sweeteners (aspartame, sucralose)
- Food colorings (like Red 40, Yellow 5)
- Preservatives (like sodium benzoate, BHT, BHA)
- Flavor enhancers (like MSG)

Breakfast Recipes

1. Spinach and Feta Omelette
Ingredients:
- 3 large eggs
- 1/4 cup crumbled feta cheese
- 1 cup fresh spinach leaves, chopped
- 1 tablespoon olive oil
- 1/4 teaspoon garlic powder
- 1/4 teaspoon dried oregano

Instructions:
1. In a medium bowl, beat the eggs until well mixed. Stir in the garlic powder and dried oregano.
2. Heat the olive oil in a non-stick skillet over medium heat.
3. Add the chopped spinach to the skillet and sauté until wilted, about 2 minutes.
4. Pour the beaten eggs into the skillet, spreading them evenly over the spinach.
5. Sprinkle the feta cheese evenly over the eggs.
6. Cook until the edges of the omelette start to set, about 2-3 minutes.
7. Gently lift the edges of the omelette with a spatula and fold it in half. Cook for another 1-2 minutes, until the eggs are fully set.
8. Slide the omelette onto a plate and serve immediately.

Nutrition Info per Serving:
- Calories: 290
- Protein: 18g
- Carbohydrates: 3g
- Fat: 22g
- Fiber: 1g

Servings:
- Serves 1

Cooking Time:
- **Total: 10 minutes**

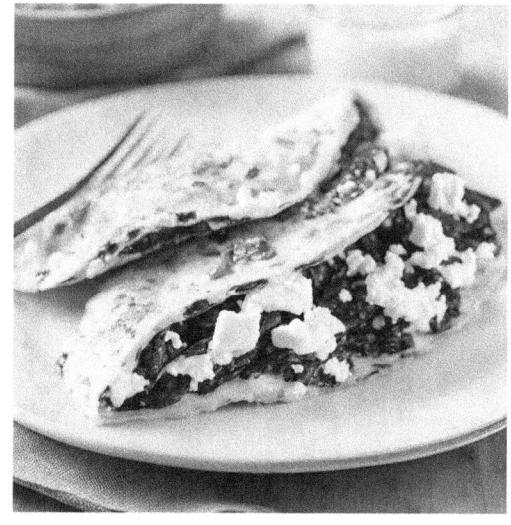

2. Greek Yogurt Parfait with Nuts and Berries

Ingredients:
- 1 cup plain Greek yogurt
- 1/2 cup mixed berries (blueberries, strawberries, raspberries)
- 2 tablespoons chopped nuts (almonds, walnuts)
- 1 tablespoon honey
- 1 teaspoon chia seeds
- 1/4 teaspoon cinnamon

Instructions:
1. In a glass or bowl, add half of the Greek yogurt.
2. Layer half of the mixed berries on top of the yogurt.
3. Sprinkle 1 tablespoon of the chopped nuts over the berries.
4. Drizzle 1/2 tablespoon of honey over the nuts.
5. Add the remaining Greek yogurt on top.
6. Top with the remaining berries and chopped nuts.
7. Sprinkle the chia seeds and cinnamon evenly over the top.
8. Serve immediately.

Nutrition Info per Serving:
- Calories: 300
- Protein: 20g
- Carbohydrates: 30g
- Fat: 12g
- Fiber: 5g

Servings:
- Serves 1

Cooking Time:
- **Total: 5 minutes**

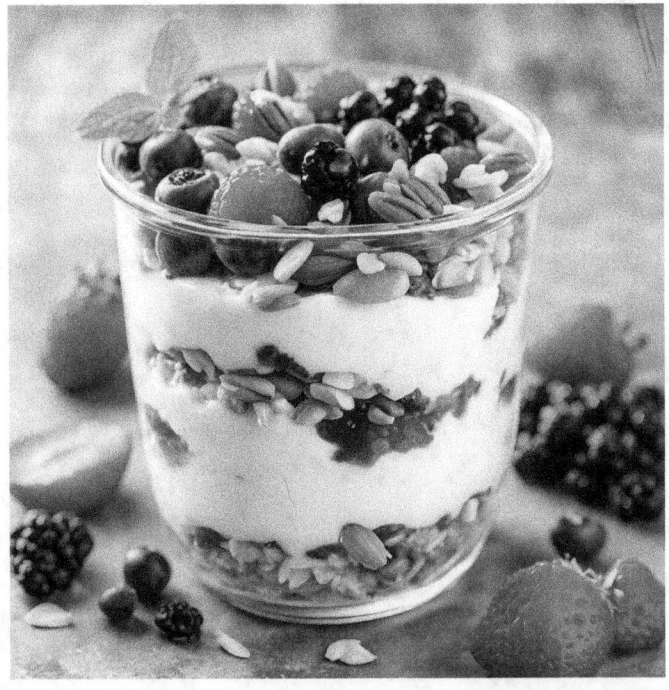

3. Almond Butter Banana Smoothie

Ingredients:
- 1 medium banana, frozen
- 1 tablespoon almond butter
- 1/2 cup unsweetened almond milk
- 1/4 cup Greek yogurt
- 1 tablespoon chia seeds
- 1/2 teaspoon vanilla extract
- 1/4 teaspoon cinnamon

Instructions:
1. In a blender, combine the frozen banana, almond butter, unsweetened almond milk, Greek yogurt, chia seeds, vanilla extract, and cinnamon.
2. Blend until smooth and creamy.
3. Pour the smoothie into a glass.
4. Serve immediately.

Nutrition Info per Serving:
- Calories: 320
- Protein: 9g
- Carbohydrates: 42g
- Fat: 14g
- Fiber: 8g

Servings:
- Serves 1

Cooking Time:
- **Total: 5 minutes**

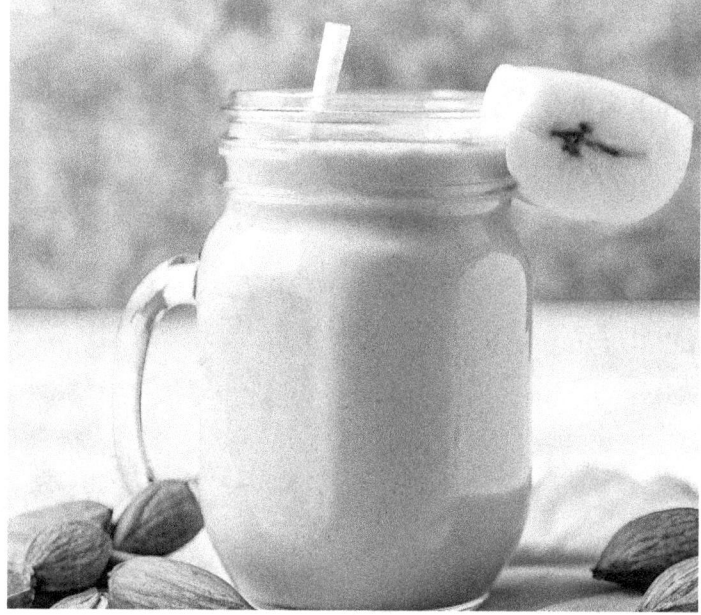

4. Turkey and Spinach Scramble

Ingredients:
- 3 large eggs
- 1/2 cup cooked turkey breast, chopped
- 1 cup fresh spinach leaves, chopped
- 1/4 cup diced bell pepper
- 1 tablespoon olive oil
- 1/4 teaspoon garlic powder
- 1/4 teaspoon paprika

Instructions:
1. In a medium bowl, beat the eggs until well mixed. Stir in the garlic powder and paprika.
2. Heat the olive oil in a non-stick skillet over medium heat.
3. Add the diced bell pepper and sauté until softened, about 3 minutes.
4. Add the chopped spinach and cook until wilted, about 2 minutes.
5. Stir in the cooked turkey breast.
6. Pour the beaten eggs into the skillet, stirring gently to combine with the turkey and vegetables.
7. Cook until the eggs are set but still moist, about 2-3 minutes.
8. Serve immediately.

Nutrition Info per Serving:
- Calories: 320
- Protein: 32g
- Carbohydrates: 5g
- Fat: 20g
- Fiber: 2g

Servings:
- Serves 1

Cooking Time:
- Total: 10 minutes

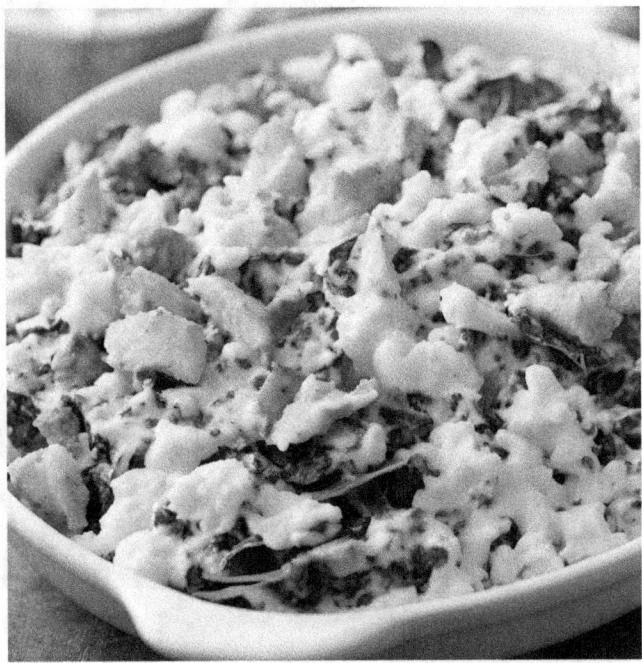

5. Protein Pancakes

Ingredients:
- 1/2 cup rolled oats
- 1/2 cup cottage cheese
- 3 large eggs
- 1/2 teaspoon baking powder
- 1/2 teaspoon vanilla extract
- 1/4 teaspoon cinnamon
- 1 tablespoon coconut oil (for cooking)

Instructions:
1. In a blender, combine the rolled oats, cottage cheese, eggs, baking powder, vanilla extract, and cinnamon. Blend until smooth.
2. Heat the coconut oil in a non-stick skillet over medium heat.
3. Pour the batter onto the skillet, forming small pancakes. Cook until bubbles form on the surface, then flip and cook until golden brown, about 2-3 minutes per side.
4. Serve immediately with your choice of toppings (e.g., fresh berries, Greek yogurt, or a drizzle of honey).

Nutrition Info per Serving:
- Calories: 350
- Protein: 28g
- Carbohydrates: 28g
- Fat: 14g
- Fiber: 4g

Servings:
- **Serves 2**

Cooking Time:
- **Total: 15 minutes**

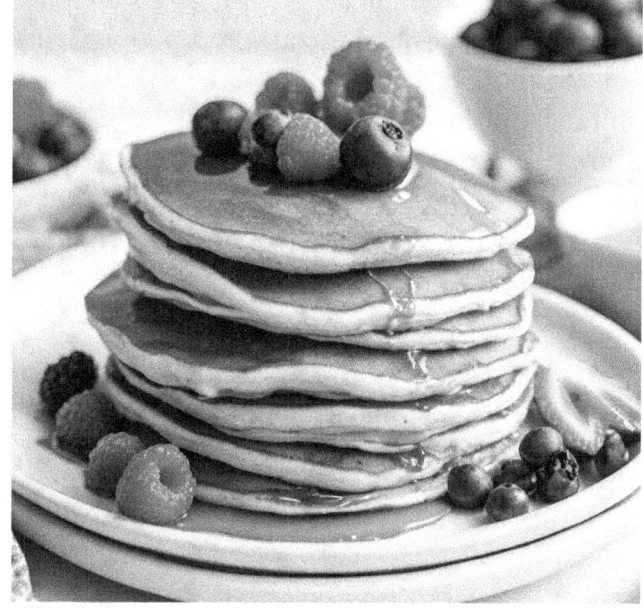

6. Vegetable Stir-Fry with Tofu

Ingredients:
- 1 block firm tofu, drained and cubed
- 2 tablespoons olive oil
- 1 cup broccoli florets
- 1 red bell pepper, sliced
- 1 cup snap peas
- 2 cloves garlic, minced
- 1 tablespoon ginger, grated
- 3 tablespoons low-sodium soy sauce
- 1 tablespoon sesame oil
- 1/2 teaspoon red pepper flakes (optional)

Instructions:
1. Heat 1 tablespoon of olive oil in a large skillet over medium-high heat.
2. Add the cubed tofu and cook until golden brown, about 5 minutes. Remove from the skillet and set aside.
3. Add the remaining olive oil to the skillet.
4. Add the broccoli, bell pepper, and snap peas. Cook for 4-5 minutes until vegetables are tender-crisp.
5. Stir in the garlic and ginger and cook for 1 minute until fragrant.
6. Return the tofu to the skillet.
7. Add the soy sauce, sesame oil, and red pepper flakes (if using). Stir to combine and cook for another 2 minutes.
8. Serve immediately.

Nutrition Info per Serving:
- Calories: 300
- Protein: 20g
- Carbohydrates: 14g
- Fat: 20g
- Fiber: 5g

Servings:
- Serves 2

Cooking Time:
- **Total: 15 minutes**

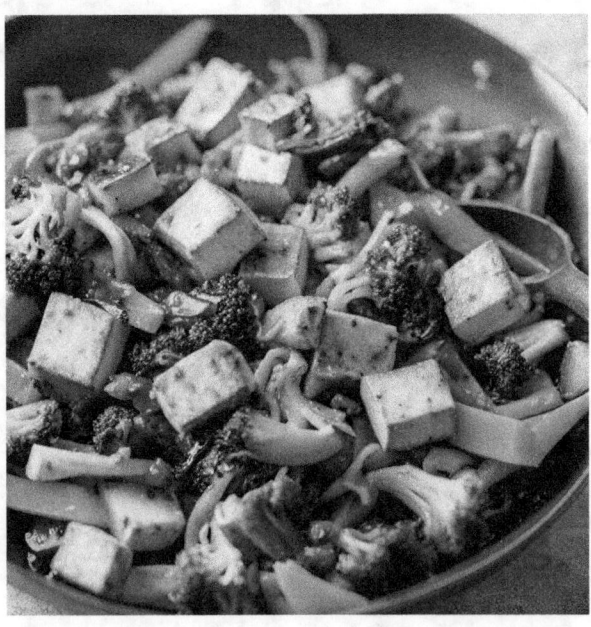

7. Quinoa Porridge

Ingredients:
- 1 cup quinoa, rinsed
- 2 cups unsweetened almond milk
- 1 cup water
- 1 teaspoon vanilla extract
- 1 teaspoon cinnamon
- 1 tablespoon maple syrup
- 1/4 cup chopped nuts (almonds, walnuts)
- 1/4 cup fresh berries (blueberries, strawberries)

Instructions:
1. In a medium saucepan, combine the quinoa, almond milk, water, vanilla extract, and cinnamon.
2. Bring to a boil, then reduce the heat to low and simmer for 15-20 minutes, until the quinoa is tender and the liquid is absorbed.
3. Stir in the maple syrup.
4. Serve the porridge topped with chopped nuts and fresh berries.

Nutrition Info per Serving:
- Calories: 350
- Protein: 10g
- Carbohydrates: 55g
- Fat: 12g
- Fiber: 7g

Servings:
- Serves 2

Cooking Time:
- **Total: 20 minutes**

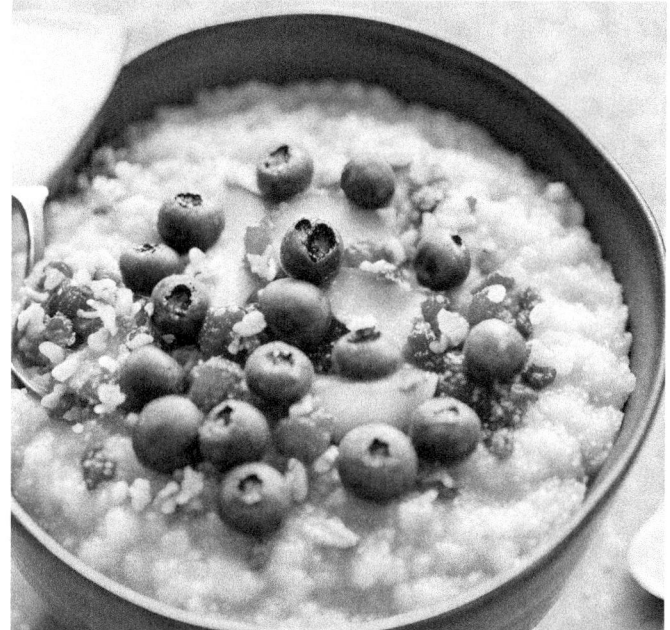

8. Egg Muffins with Veggies and Cheese

Ingredients:
- 6 large eggs
- 1/2 cup shredded cheddar cheese
- 1/2 cup diced bell pepper
- 1/2 cup chopped spinach
- 1/4 cup diced onion
- 1/4 cup milk
- 1/4 teaspoon garlic powder
- 1/4 teaspoon dried oregano

Instructions:
1. Preheat the oven to 350°F (175°C).
2. In a large bowl, beat the eggs and milk until well combined. Stir in the garlic powder and dried oregano.
3. Fold in the diced bell pepper, chopped spinach, and diced onion.
4. Grease a muffin tin with cooking spray or olive oil.
5. Pour the egg mixture evenly into the muffin cups, filling them about 3/4 full.
6. Sprinkle the shredded cheddar cheese on top of each muffin.
7. Bake for 20-25 minutes, until the muffins are set and golden brown.
8. Allow to cool slightly before removing from the muffin tin. Serve warm.

Nutrition Info per Serving:
- Calories: 150
- Protein: 12g
- Carbohydrates: 3g
- Fat: 10g
- Fiber: 1g

Servings:
- Serves 6

Cooking Time:
- Total: 30 minutes

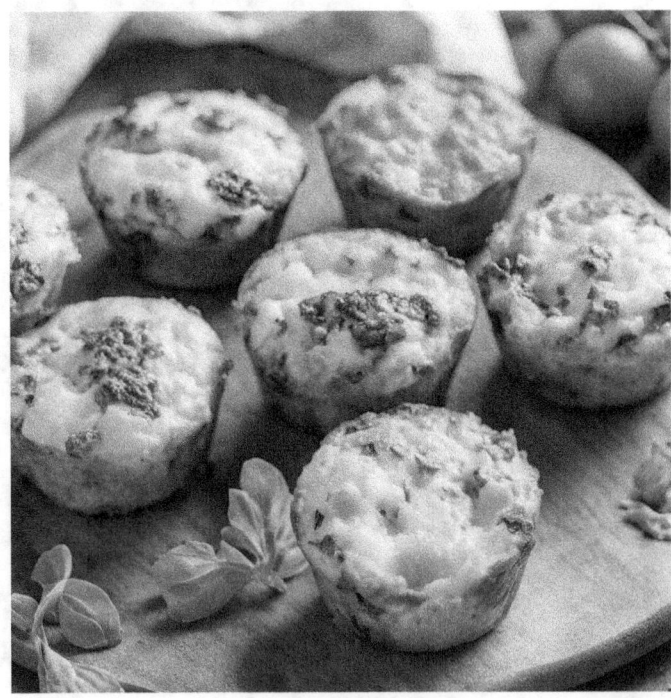

9. Kale and Sweet Potato Hash

Ingredients:
- 2 medium sweet potatoes, peeled and diced
- 1 cup chopped kale
- 1 small onion, diced
- 2 cloves garlic, minced
- 1 tablespoon olive oil
- 1/2 teaspoon smoked paprika
- 1/4 teaspoon cumin

Instructions:
1. Heat the olive oil in a large skillet over medium heat.
2. Add the diced sweet potatoes and cook until they begin to soften, about 10 minutes.
3. Add the diced onion and garlic, cooking until the onion is translucent, about 5 minutes.
4. Stir in the chopped kale, smoked paprika, and cumin. Cook until the kale is wilted and sweet potatoes are tender, about 5 more minutes.
5. Serve immediately.

Nutrition Info per Serving:
- Calories: 200
- Protein: 3g
- Carbohydrates: 30g
- Fat: 7g
- Fiber: 6g

Servings:
- Serves 2

Cooking Time:
- **Total: 20 minutes**

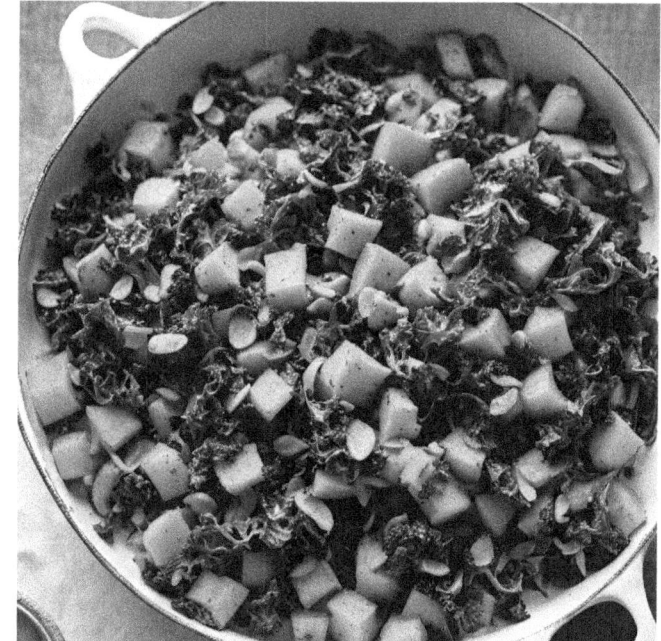

10. Low Carb Blueberry Muffins

Ingredients:
- 2 cups almond flour
- 1/4 cup coconut flour
- 1/2 cup blueberries
- 3 large eggs
- 1/3 cup unsweetened almond milk
- 1/4 cup melted coconut oil
- 1/4 cup honey
- 1 teaspoon baking powder
- 1 teaspoon vanilla extract
- 1/2 teaspoon cinnamon

Instructions:
1. Preheat the oven to 350°F (175°C) and line a muffin tin with paper liners.
2. In a large bowl, whisk together the almond flour, coconut flour, baking powder, and cinnamon.
3. In another bowl, beat the eggs, almond milk, melted coconut oil, honey, and vanilla extract until well combined.
4. Add the wet ingredients to the dry ingredients and mix until just combined.
5. Gently fold in the blueberries.
6. Divide the batter evenly among the muffin cups.
7. Bake for 20-25 minutes, or until a toothpick inserted into the center comes out clean.
8. Allow to cool before serving.

Nutrition Info per Serving:
- Calories: 180
- Protein: 5g
- Carbohydrates: 12g
- Fat: 14g
- Fiber: 3g

Servings:
- **Serves 12**

Cooking Time:
- **Total: 30 minutes**

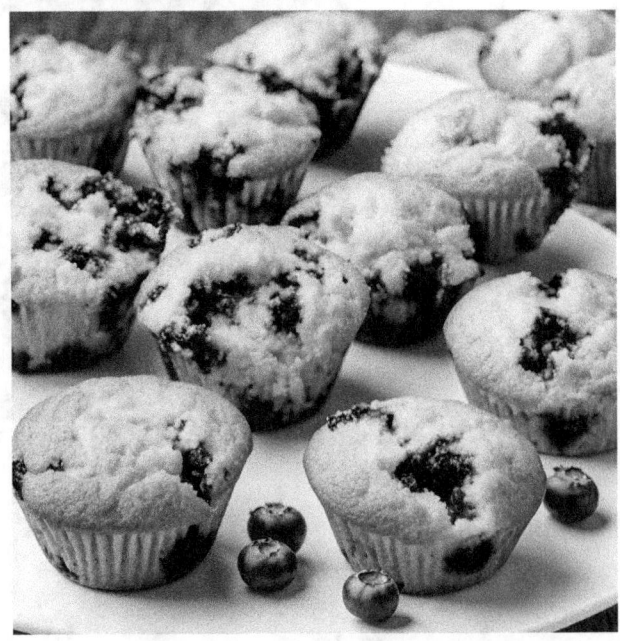

11. Zucchini and Carrot Fritters

Ingredients:
- 1 medium zucchini, grated
- 1 medium carrot, grated
- 1/4 cup almond flour
- 2 large eggs, beaten
- 2 tablespoons chopped fresh parsley
- 1 clove garlic, minced
- 1/4 teaspoon paprika
- 2 tablespoons olive oil

Instructions:
1. Place the grated zucchini and carrot in a clean kitchen towel and squeeze out excess moisture.
2. In a large bowl, combine the zucchini, carrot, almond flour, beaten eggs, parsley, garlic, and paprika. Mix well.
3. Heat the olive oil in a large skillet over medium heat.
4. Scoop 1/4 cup of the mixture for each fritter and place in the skillet, flattening with a spatula.
5. Cook for 3-4 minutes on each side, until golden brown.
6. Remove from the skillet and drain on paper towels. Serve warm.

Nutrition Info per Serving:
- Calories: 120
- Protein: 4g
- Carbohydrates: 6g
- Fat: 9g
- Fiber: 2g

Servings:
- Serves 4

Cooking Time:
- **Total: 20 minutes**

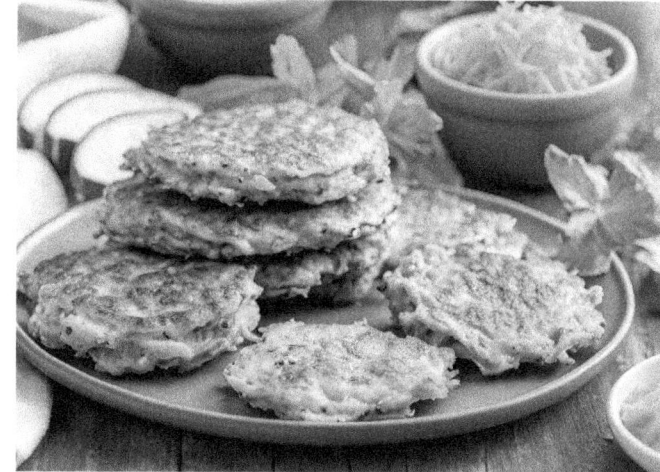

12. Overnight Oats with Flaxseed

Ingredients:
- 1/2 cup rolled oats
- 1 tablespoon flaxseed meal
- 1/2 cup unsweetened almond milk
- 1/4 cup Greek yogurt
- 1 tablespoon honey
- 1/4 teaspoon cinnamon
- 1/4 cup fresh berries (optional)

Instructions:
1. In a mason jar or bowl, combine the rolled oats, flaxseed meal, almond milk, Greek yogurt, honey, and cinnamon. Stir well.
2. Cover and refrigerate overnight.
3. In the morning, stir the oats and top with fresh berries if desired. Serve cold.

Nutrition Info per Serving:
- Calories: 250
- Protein: 10g
- Carbohydrates: 35g
- Fat: 8g
- Fiber: 6g

Servings:
- Serves 1

Cooking Time:
- **Total: 5 minutes prep, overnight refrigeration**

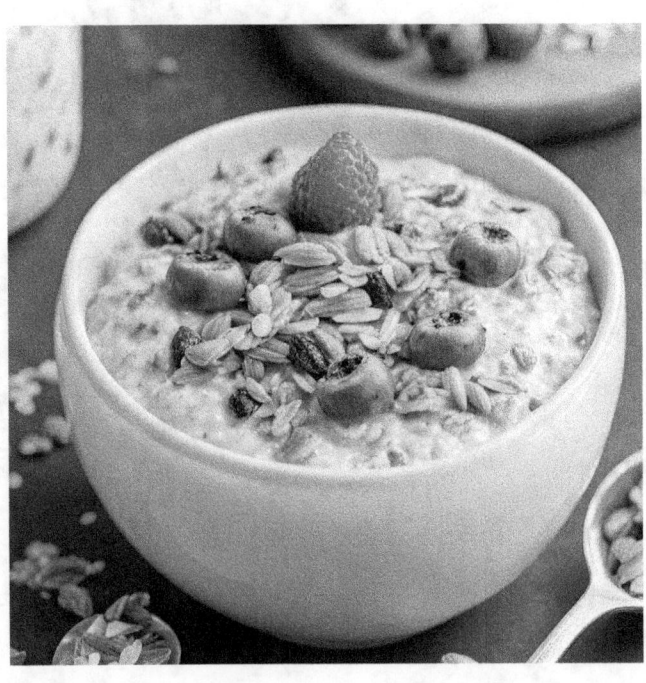

13. Chicken Sausage Breakfast Burrito

Ingredients:
- 2 chicken sausages, cooked and sliced
- 2 large eggs
- 1/4 cup shredded cheddar cheese
- 1/2 cup diced bell pepper
- 1/4 cup diced onion
- 1 tablespoon olive oil
- 2 whole grain tortillas
- 1/4 teaspoon garlic powder
- 1/4 teaspoon cumin

Instructions:
1. Heat the olive oil in a skillet over medium heat.
2. Add the diced bell pepper and onion, cooking until softened, about 5 minutes.
3. Add the sliced chicken sausages and cook until heated through.
4. In a bowl, beat the eggs with the garlic powder and cumin, then pour into the skillet.
5. Cook the eggs, stirring constantly, until set.
6. Warm the tortillas in a separate skillet or microwave.
7. Divide the egg mixture between the tortillas, sprinkle with shredded cheddar cheese, and roll up the burritos.
8. Serve immediately.

Nutrition Info per Serving:
- Calories: 350
- Protein: 20g
- Carbohydrates: 25g
- Fat: 18g
- Fiber: 5g

Servings:
- Serves 2

Cooking Time:
- **Total: 15 minutes**

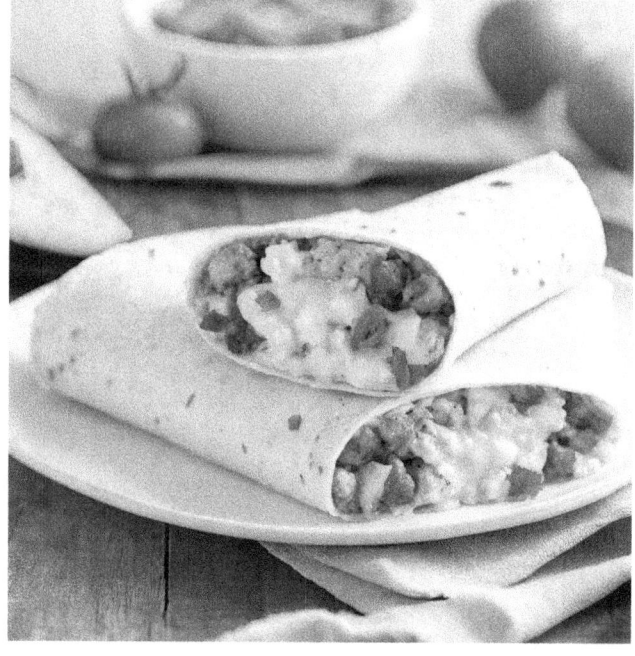

14. Pumpkin Seed Granola

Ingredients:
- 2 cups rolled oats
- 1/2 cup pumpkin seeds
- 1/2 cup chopped almonds
- 1/4 cup chia seeds
- 1/4 cup honey
- 1/4 cup melted coconut oil
- 1 teaspoon vanilla extract
- 1/2 teaspoon cinnamon

Instructions:
1. Preheat the oven to 300°F (150°C).
2. In a large bowl, mix the rolled oats, pumpkin seeds, chopped almonds, and chia seeds.
3. In a small saucepan over low heat, combine the honey, melted coconut oil, vanilla extract, and cinnamon. Stir until well combined.
4. Pour the honey mixture over the dry ingredients and stir until everything is evenly coated.
5. Spread the mixture evenly on a baking sheet lined with parchment paper.
6. Bake for 25-30 minutes, stirring halfway through, until golden brown.
7. Allow to cool completely before storing in an airtight container.

Nutrition Info per Serving:
- Calories: 250
- Protein: 6g
- Carbohydrates: 30g
- Fat: 12g
- Fiber: 5g

Servings:
- **Serves 8**

Cooking Time:
- **Total: 35 minutes**

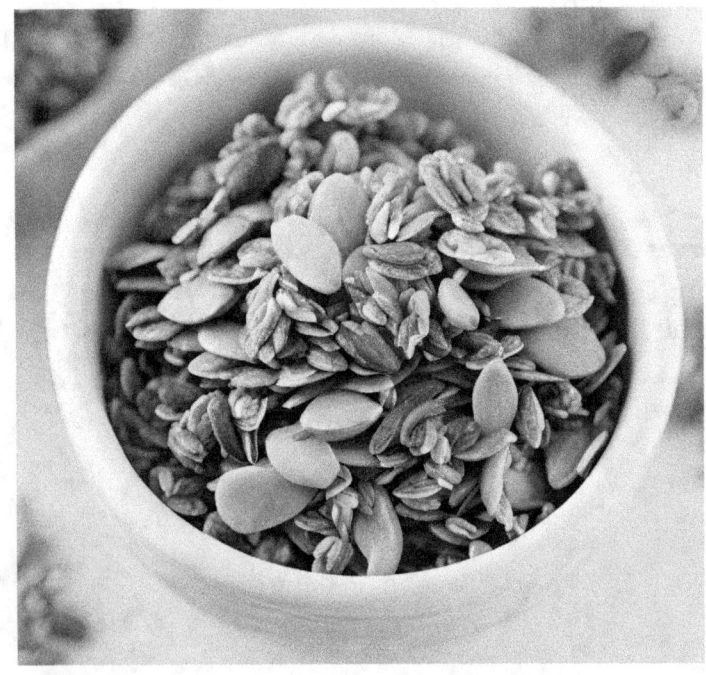

15. Soy and Linseed Porridge

Ingredients:
- 1/2 cup rolled oats
- 1 cup unsweetened soy milk
- 1 tablespoon linseeds (flaxseeds)
- 1 teaspoon honey
- 1/4 teaspoon cinnamon
- 1/4 cup fresh berries (optional)

Instructions:
1. In a medium saucepan, combine the rolled oats, unsweetened soy milk, linseeds, and cinnamon.
2. Bring to a boil over medium heat, then reduce the heat to low and simmer for 5-7 minutes, stirring occasionally, until the oats are tender and the porridge is thick.
3. Stir in the honey.
4. Serve topped with fresh berries if desired.

Nutrition Info per Serving:
- Calories: 220
- Protein: 8g
- Carbohydrates: 35g
- Fat: 6g
- Fiber: 7g

Servings:
- Serves 1

Cooking Time:
- **Total: 10 minutes**

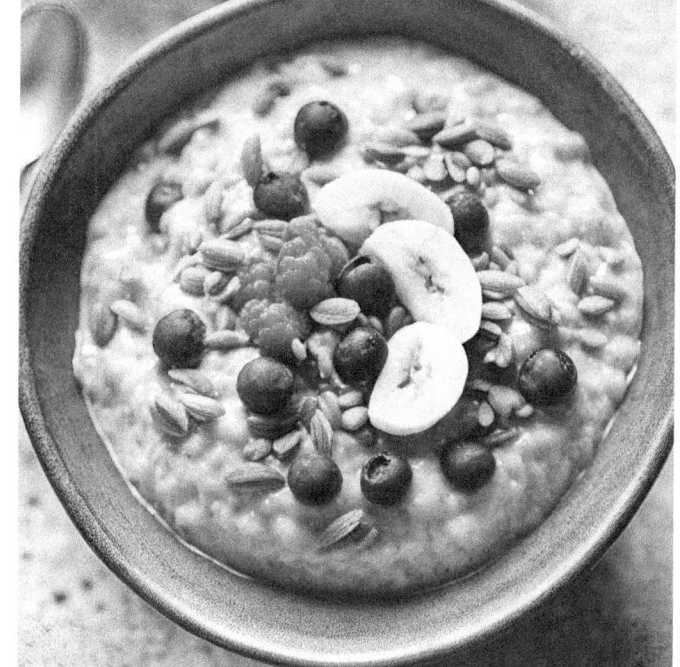

16. Buckwheat Pancakes

Ingredients:
- 1 cup buckwheat flour
- 1 cup unsweetened almond milk
- 1 large egg
- 1 tablespoon melted coconut oil
- 1 tablespoon honey
- 1 teaspoon baking powder
- 1/2 teaspoon vanilla extract
- 1/4 teaspoon cinnamon

Instructions:
1. In a large bowl, whisk together the buckwheat flour, baking powder, and cinnamon.
2. In another bowl, beat the egg and then add the almond milk, melted coconut oil, honey, and vanilla extract. Mix well.
3. Pour the wet ingredients into the dry ingredients and stir until just combined.
4. Heat a non-stick skillet over medium heat and lightly grease with a small amount of coconut oil.
5. Pour 1/4 cup of batter onto the skillet for each pancake. Cook until bubbles form on the surface, then flip and cook until golden brown, about 2-3 minutes per side.
6. Serve immediately with your choice of toppings (e.g., fresh fruit, Greek yogurt, or a drizzle of honey).

Nutrition Info per Serving:
- Calories: 180
- Protein: 5g
- Carbohydrates: 28g
- Fat: 6g
- Fiber: 4g

Servings:
- Serves 4

Cooking Time:
- **Total: 20 minutes**

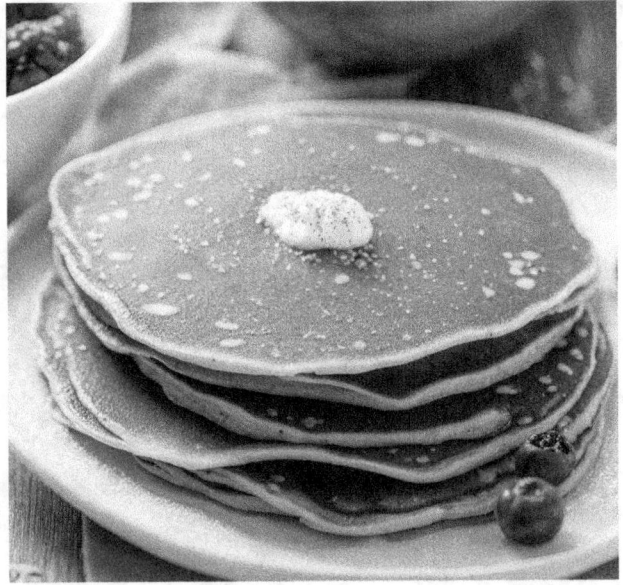

17. Beetroot and Ginger Smoothie

Ingredients:
- 1 medium beetroot, cooked and peeled
- 1 medium banana
- 1/2 cup unsweetened almond milk
- 1/4 cup Greek yogurt
- 1 tablespoon chia seeds
- 1/2 teaspoon grated fresh ginger
- 1 tablespoon honey

Instructions:
1. In a blender, combine the cooked beetroot, banana, unsweetened almond milk, Greek yogurt, chia seeds, grated ginger, and honey.
2. Blend until smooth and creamy.
3. Pour the smoothie into a glass.
4. Serve immediately.

Nutrition Info per Serving:
- Calories: 220   Protein: 6g   Carbohydrates: 42g   Fat: 5g   Fiber: 8g
- **Servings:**   Serves 1

Cooking Time: Total: 5 minutes

18. Tuna Salad on Whole Wheat Toast

Ingredients:
- 1 can (5 oz) tuna in water, drained
- 2 tablespoons Greek yogurt
- 1 tablespoon diced celery
- 1 tablespoon diced red onion
- 1 teaspoon lemon juice
- 1/4 teaspoon dried dill
- 2 slices whole wheat bread, toasted

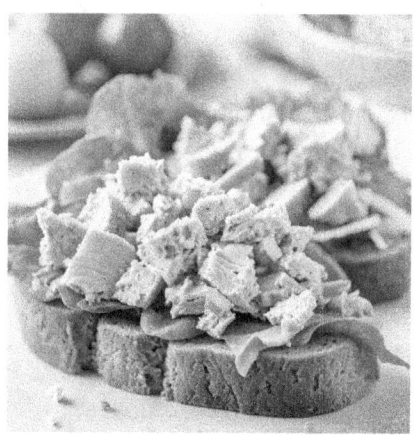

Instructions:
1. In a medium bowl, combine the drained tuna, Greek yogurt, diced celery, diced red onion, lemon juice, and dried dill. Mix well.
2. Toast the whole wheat bread slices.
3. Spread the tuna salad evenly over the toasted bread slices.
4. Serve immediately.

Nutrition Info per Serving:
- Calories: 300   Protein: 25g   Carbohydrates: 30g   Fat: 10g   Fiber: 5g

Servings: Serves 1

Cooking Time:
- **Total: 10 minutes**

19. Asparagus and Mushroom Frittata

Ingredients:
- 6 large eggs
- 1/2 cup unsweetened almond milk
- 1 cup asparagus, trimmed and cut into 1-inch pieces
- 1 cup sliced mushrooms
- 1/2 cup shredded mozzarella cheese
- 1 tablespoon olive oil
- 1/2 teaspoon garlic powder
- 1/4 teaspoon dried thyme

Instructions:
1. Preheat the oven to 350°F (175°C).
2. In a large bowl, whisk together the eggs, almond milk, garlic powder, and dried thyme.
3. Heat the olive oil in an oven-safe skillet over medium heat.
4. Add the asparagus and mushrooms, cooking until tender, about 5-7 minutes.
5. Pour the egg mixture over the vegetables in the skillet and cook for 2-3 minutes, until the edges begin to set.
6. Sprinkle the shredded mozzarella cheese on top.
7. Transfer the skillet to the oven and bake for 15-20 minutes, until the frittata is fully set and golden brown.
8. Remove from the oven and let cool slightly before slicing and serving.

Nutrition Info per Serving:
- Calories: 180
- Protein: 15g
- Carbohydrates: 5g
- Fat: 12g
- Fiber: 2g

Servings:
- Serves 4

Cooking Time:
- **Total: 30 minutes**

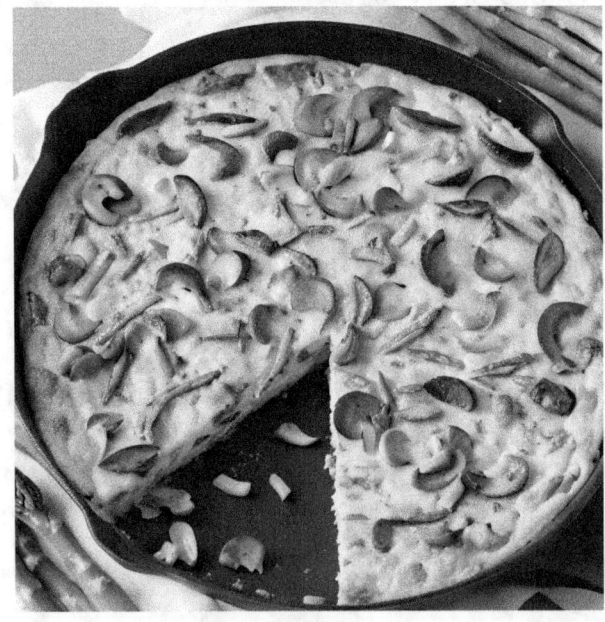

20. Muesli with Skim Milk

Ingredients:
- 1 cup rolled oats
- 1/4 cup chopped almonds
- 1/4 cup raisins
- 1/4 cup sunflower seeds
- 1/2 teaspoon cinnamon
- 1 cup skim milk
- 1/2 cup fresh berries (optional)

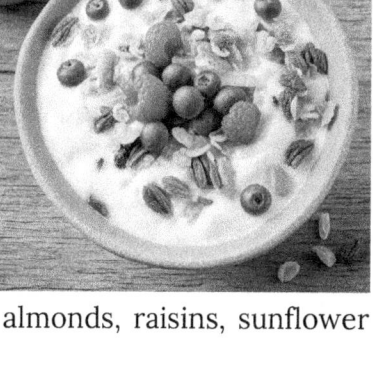

Instructions:
1. In a large bowl, combine the rolled oats, chopped almonds, raisins, sunflower seeds, and cinnamon.
2. Divide the muesli mixture into bowls.
3. Pour 1/2 cup of skim milk over each serving.
4. Top with fresh berries if desired.
5. Serve immediately or refrigerate overnight for a softer texture.

Nutrition Info per Serving:
- Calories: 250   Protein: 8g   Carbohydrates: 40g   Fat: 8g   Fiber: 6g

Servings: Serves 2
Cooking Time: Total: 5 minutes

21. Protein-Packed Lentil Salad

Ingredients:
- 1 cup cooked green lentils
- 1/2 cup cherry tomatoes, halved
- 1/4 cup diced cucumber
- 1/4 cup crumbled feta cheese
- 2 tablespoons chopped fresh parsley
- 1 tablespoon olive oil
- 1 tablespoon lemon juice
- 1/2 teaspoon dried oregano

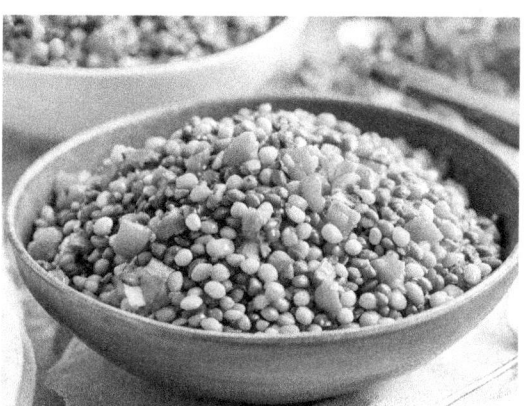

Instructions:
1. In a large bowl, combine the cooked lentils, cherry tomatoes, cucumber, feta cheese, and parsley.
2. In a small bowl, whisk together the olive oil, lemon juice, and dried oregano.
3. Pour the dressing over the lentil mixture and toss to combine.
4. Serve immediately or refrigerate until ready to eat.

Nutrition Info per Serving:
- Calories: 280   Protein: 14g   Carbohydrates: 30g   Fat: 12g   Fiber: 10g

Servings: Serves 2
Cooking Time: Total: 10 minutes

22. Sweet Potato and Black Bean Breakfast Bowl

Ingredients:
- 1 medium sweet potato, peeled and diced
- 1/2 cup black beans, drained and rinsed
- 1/2 avocado, sliced
- 1/4 cup diced red bell pepper
- 1 tablespoon olive oil
- 1/4 teaspoon cumin
- 1/4 teaspoon smoked paprika
- 1 tablespoon chopped fresh cilantro (optional)

Instructions:
1. Preheat the oven to 400°F (200°C).
2. Toss the diced sweet potato with olive oil, cumin, and smoked paprika. Spread in a single layer on a baking sheet.
3. Roast the sweet potato in the oven for 20-25 minutes, until tender and slightly crispy.
4. In a bowl, combine the roasted sweet potato, black beans, red bell pepper, and avocado slices.
5. Sprinkle with chopped fresh cilantro if desired.
6. Serve immediately.

Nutrition Info per Serving:
- Calories: 350
- Protein: 8g
- Carbohydrates: 45g
- Fat: 18g
- Fiber: 12g

Servings: Serves 2
Cooking Time: Total: 30 minutes

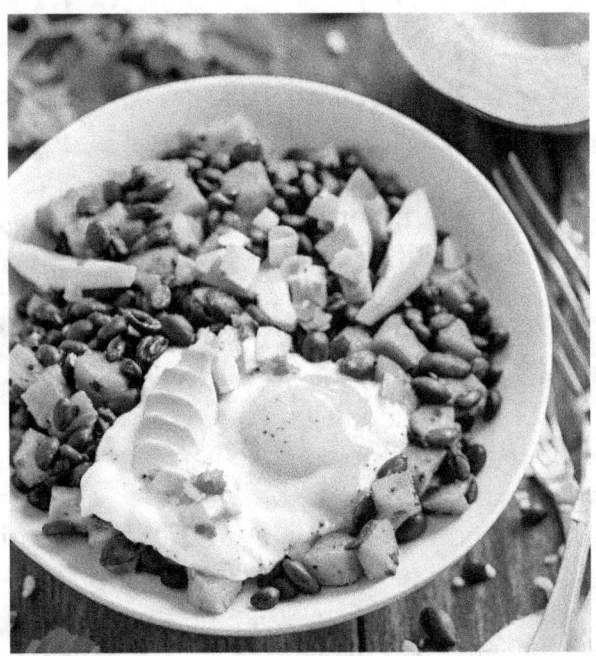

23. Tempeh and Broccoli Sauté

Ingredients:
- 1 block tempeh, cut into cubes
- 2 cups broccoli florets
- 1 red bell pepper, sliced
- 2 tablespoons olive oil
- 2 cloves garlic, minced
- 1 tablespoon low-sodium soy sauce
- 1 teaspoon grated ginger
- 1/4 teaspoon red pepper flakes (optional)

Instructions:
1. Heat 1 tablespoon of olive oil in a large skillet over medium heat.
2. Add the tempeh cubes and cook until golden brown on all sides, about 5-7 minutes. Remove from the skillet and set aside.
3. Add the remaining tablespoon of olive oil to the skillet.
4. Add the broccoli florets and red bell pepper slices. Cook until tender-crisp, about 5 minutes.
5. Stir in the minced garlic, grated ginger, and red pepper flakes (if using), and cook for another 1-2 minutes.
6. Return the tempeh to the skillet and add the soy sauce. Stir to combine and heat through.
7. Serve immediately.

Nutrition Info per Serving:
- Calories: 250
- Protein: 15g
- Carbohydrates: 20g
- Fat: 12g
- Fiber: 5g

Servings:
- Serves 2

Cooking Time:
- **Total: 15 minutes**

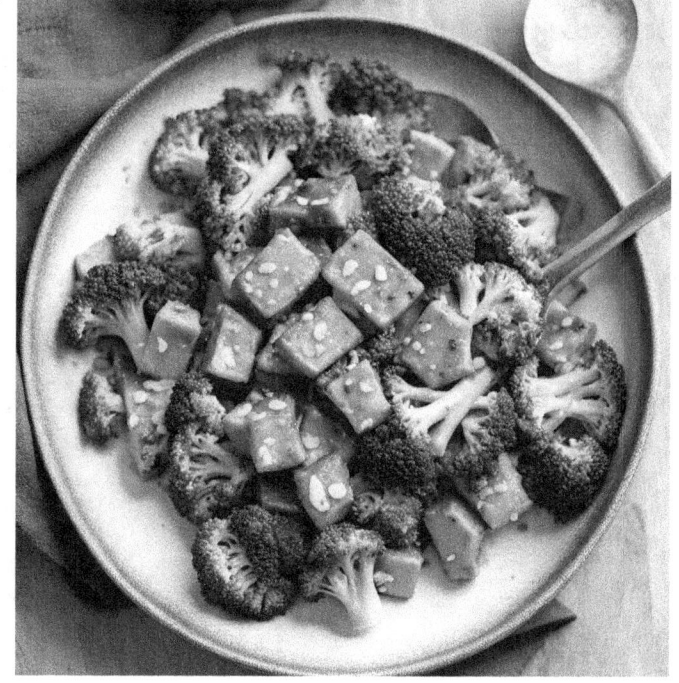

24. Almond Flour Waffles

Ingredients:
- 2 cups almond flour
- 3 large eggs
- 1/4 cup unsweetened almond milk
- 2 tablespoons melted coconut oil
- 1 tablespoon honey
- 1 teaspoon baking powder
- 1/2 teaspoon vanilla extract
- 1/4 teaspoon cinnamon

Instructions:
1. Preheat your waffle iron according to the manufacturer's instructions.
2. In a large bowl, whisk together the almond flour, baking powder, and cinnamon.
3. In another bowl, beat the eggs and then add the almond milk, melted coconut oil, honey, and vanilla extract. Mix well.
4. Pour the wet ingredients into the dry ingredients and stir until just combined.
5. Lightly grease the waffle iron with coconut oil or cooking spray.
6. Pour the batter into the waffle iron and cook according to the manufacturer's instructions, usually 3-5 minutes, until golden brown.
7. Serve immediately with your choice of toppings (e.g., fresh berries, Greek yogurt, or a drizzle of honey).

Nutrition Info per Serving:
- Calories: 350
- Protein: 12g
- Carbohydrates: 12g
- Fat: 28g
- Fiber: 5g

Servings:
- Serves 4

Cooking Time:
- **Total: 15 minutes**

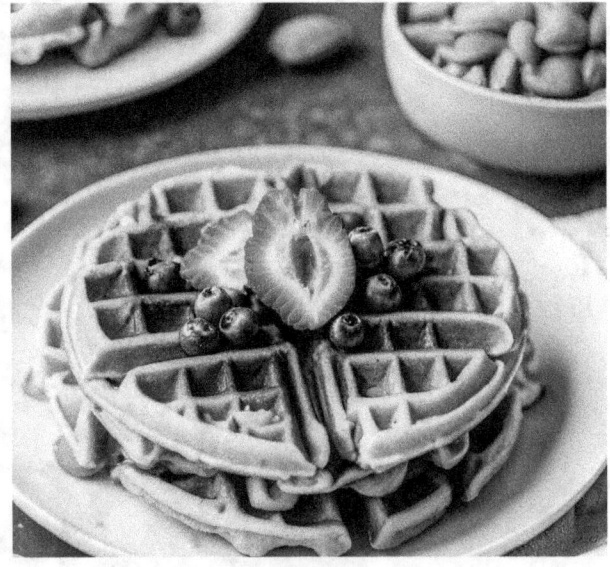

25. Oat Bran Muffin

Ingredients:
- 1 cup oat bran
- 1/2 cup whole wheat flour
- 1/2 cup unsweetened applesauce
- 1/2 cup skim milk
- 1/4 cup honey
- 2 large eggs
- 1 teaspoon baking powder
- 1/2 teaspoon baking soda
- 1/2 teaspoon cinnamon
- 1/4 cup raisins (optional)

Instructions:
1. Preheat the oven to 375°F (190°C) and line a muffin tin with paper liners.
2. In a large bowl, combine the oat bran, whole wheat flour, baking powder, baking soda, and cinnamon.
3. In another bowl, beat the eggs and then add the unsweetened applesauce, skim milk, and honey. Mix well.
4. Pour the wet ingredients into the dry ingredients and stir until just combined.
5. Fold in the raisins if using.
6. Divide the batter evenly among the muffin cups.
7. Bake for 15-20 minutes, or until a toothpick inserted into the center comes out clean.
8. Allow to cool before serving.

Nutrition Info per Serving:
- Calories: 150
- Protein: 5g
- Carbohydrates: 28g
- Fat: 3g
- Fiber: 4g

Servings:
- Serves 12

Cooking Time:
- **Total: 25 minutes**

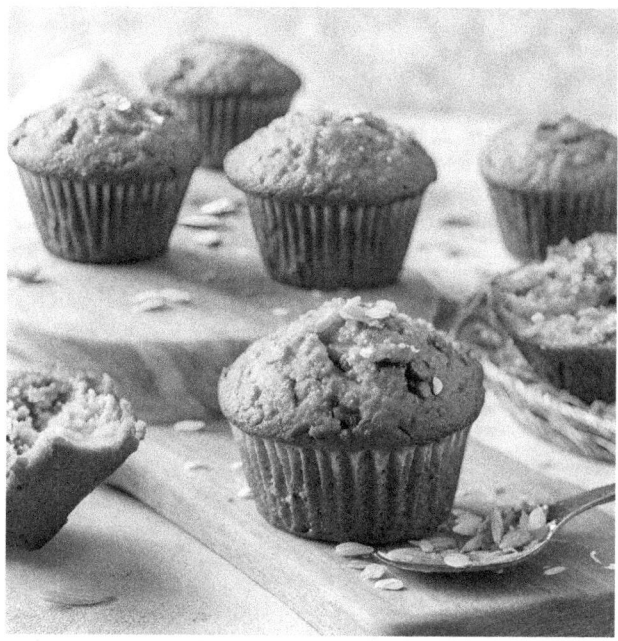

Poultry Recipes

1. Grilled Chicken with Avocado Salsa
Ingredients:
- 2 boneless, skinless chicken breasts
- 1 tablespoon olive oil
- 1 teaspoon garlic powder
- 1 teaspoon paprika
- 1 avocado, diced
- 1 small tomato, diced
- 1/4 cup red onion, finely chopped
- 1 tablespoon lime juice
- 2 tablespoons chopped fresh cilantro

Instructions:
1. Preheat the grill to medium-high heat.
2. Rub the chicken breasts with olive oil, garlic powder, and paprika.
3. Grill the chicken breasts for 6-7 minutes on each side, or until fully cooked and the internal temperature reaches 165°F (75°C).
4. While the chicken is grilling, prepare the avocado salsa. In a medium bowl, combine the diced avocado, tomato, red onion, lime juice, and cilantro. Mix gently.
5. Once the chicken is done, let it rest for a few minutes before slicing.
6. Top the grilled chicken with the avocado salsa.
7. Serve immediately.

Nutrition Info per Serving:
- Calories: 350
- Protein: 30g
- Carbohydrates: 10g
- Fat: 22g
- Fiber: 7g

Servings:
- Serves 2

Cooking Time:
- Total: 20 minutes

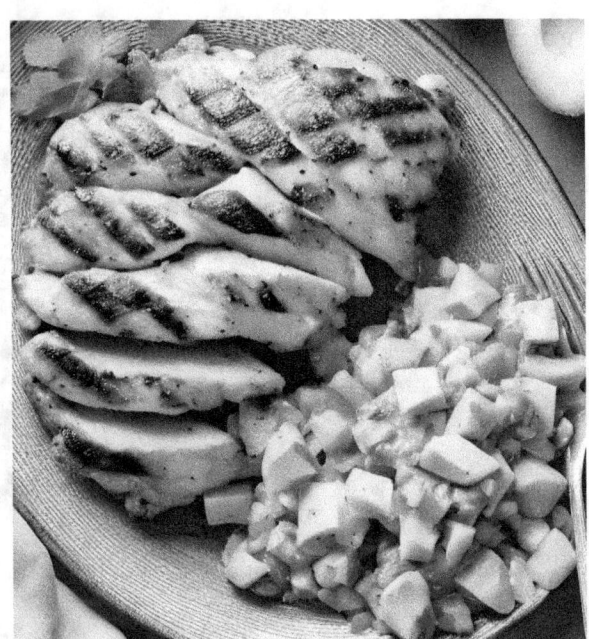

2. Turkey Lettuce Wraps

Ingredients:
- 1 pound ground turkey
- 1 tablespoon olive oil
- 1 small onion, diced
- 2 cloves garlic, minced
- 1 red bell pepper, diced
- 1/4 cup low-sodium soy sauce
- 1 tablespoon hoisin sauce
- 1 teaspoon grated ginger
- 1/4 teaspoon red pepper flakes (optional)
- 1 head butter lettuce, leaves separated

Instructions:
1. Heat the olive oil in a large skillet over medium heat.
2. Add the diced onion and cook until translucent, about 3-4 minutes.
3. Add the minced garlic and grated ginger, cooking for another minute until fragrant.
4. Add the ground turkey to the skillet, breaking it up with a spoon as it cooks. Cook until browned and fully cooked, about 5-7 minutes.
5. Stir in the diced red bell pepper, soy sauce, hoisin sauce, and red pepper flakes (if using). Cook for another 2-3 minutes until the bell pepper is tender.
6. Remove from heat and let cool slightly.
7. Spoon the turkey mixture into lettuce leaves.
8. Serve immediately.

Nutrition Info per Serving:
- Calories: 250
- Protein: 26g
- Carbohydrates: 10g
- Fat: 12g
- Fiber: 2g

Servings:
- Serves 4

Cooking Time:
- **Total: 20 minutes**

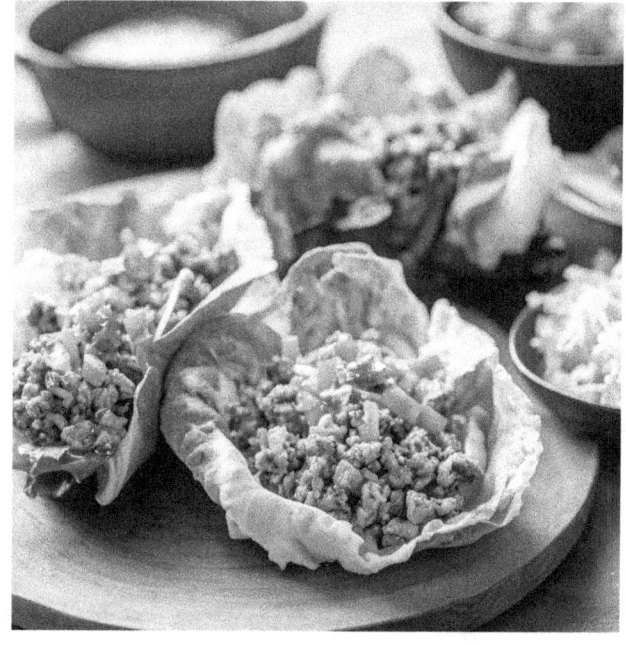

3. Chicken and Vegetable Stir-Fry

Ingredients:
- 2 boneless, skinless chicken breasts, cut into thin strips
- 2 tablespoons olive oil
- 2 cups broccoli florets
- 1 red bell pepper, sliced
- 1 yellow bell pepper, sliced
- 1 cup snap peas
- 2 cloves garlic, minced
- 1 tablespoon grated ginger
- 1/4 cup low-sodium soy sauce
- 1 tablespoon hoisin sauce
- 1 teaspoon sesame oil

Instructions:
1. Heat 1 tablespoon of olive oil in a large skillet or wok over medium-high heat.
2. Add the chicken strips and cook until browned and fully cooked, about 5-7 minutes. Remove from the skillet and set aside.
3. Add the remaining tablespoon of olive oil to the skillet.
4. Add the broccoli, red bell pepper, yellow bell pepper, and snap peas. Cook, stirring frequently, until the vegetables are tender-crisp, about 5-7 minutes.
5. Stir in the minced garlic and grated ginger, cooking for another 1-2 minutes until fragrant.
6. Return the chicken to the skillet.
7. Stir in the soy sauce, hoisin sauce, and sesame oil. Cook for another 2-3 minutes, until everything is well combined and heated through.
8. Serve immediately.

Nutrition Info per Serving:
- Calories: 300
- Protein: 28g
- Carbohydrates: 15g
- Fat: 14g
- Fiber: 5g

Servings:
- Serves 4

Cooking Time:
- **Total: 20 minutes**

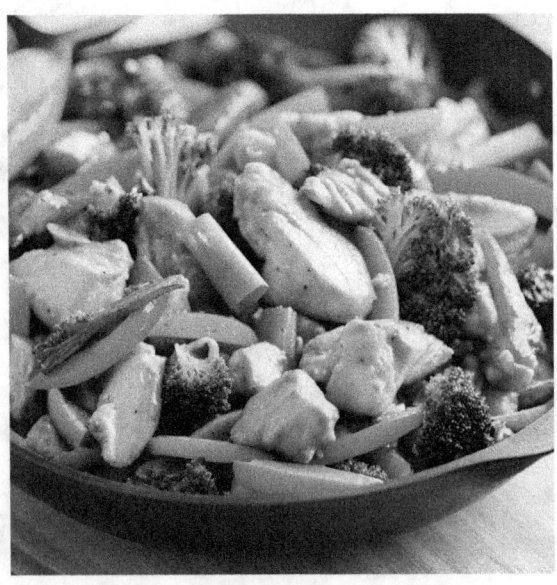

4. Baked Lemon Herb Chicken

Ingredients:
- 4 boneless, skinless chicken breasts
- 2 tablespoons olive oil
- 1 tablespoon lemon juice
- 1 teaspoon lemon zest
- 2 cloves garlic, minced
- 1 teaspoon dried oregano
- 1 teaspoon dried thyme
- 1/2 teaspoon paprika

Instructions:
1. Preheat the oven to 375°F (190°C).
2. In a small bowl, combine the olive oil, lemon juice, lemon zest, minced garlic, oregano, thyme, and paprika.
3. Place the chicken breasts in a baking dish.
4. Brush the lemon herb mixture over the chicken breasts, ensuring they are well coated.
5. Bake for 25-30 minutes, or until the chicken is fully cooked and reaches an internal temperature of 165°F (75°C).
6. Remove from the oven and let rest for a few minutes before serving.

Nutrition Info per Serving:
- Calories: 220
- Protein: 28g
- Carbohydrates: 2g
- Fat: 11g
- Fiber: 0g

Servings:
- Serves 4

Cooking Time:
- **Total: 35 minutes**

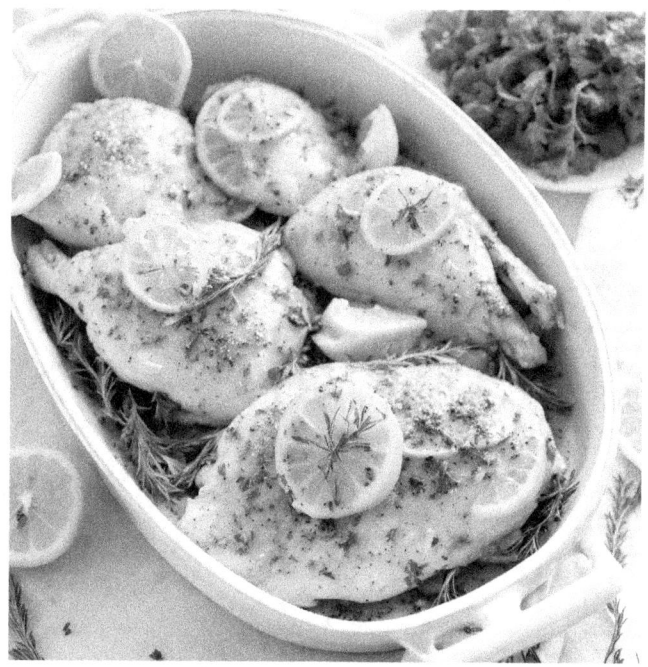

5. Ground Turkey Stuffed Peppers

Ingredients:
- 4 large bell peppers, tops cut off and seeds removed
- 1 pound ground turkey
- 1 tablespoon olive oil
- 1 small onion, diced
- 2 cloves garlic, minced
- 1 cup cooked quinoa
- 1 cup diced tomatoes
- 1 teaspoon dried oregano
- 1 teaspoon cumin
- 1/2 cup shredded mozzarella cheese

Instructions:
1. Preheat the oven to 375°F (190°C).
2. In a large skillet, heat the olive oil over medium heat.
3. Add the diced onion and cook until translucent, about 3-4 minutes.
4. Add the minced garlic and cook for another minute until fragrant.
5. Add the ground turkey and cook until browned and fully cooked, about 5-7 minutes.
6. Stir in the cooked quinoa, diced tomatoes, oregano, and cumin. Cook for another 2-3 minutes until well combined.
7. Place the bell peppers upright in a baking dish.
8. Spoon the turkey mixture into the bell peppers, filling them to the top.
9. Sprinkle the shredded mozzarella cheese on top of each stuffed pepper.
10. Bake for 25-30 minutes, until the peppers are tender and the cheese is melted and golden.
11. Serve immediately.

Nutrition Info per Serving:
- Calories: 300
- Protein: 25g
- Carbohydrates: 25g
- Fat: 12g
- Fiber: 5g

Servings:
- Serves 4

Cooking Time:
- **Total: 45 minutes**

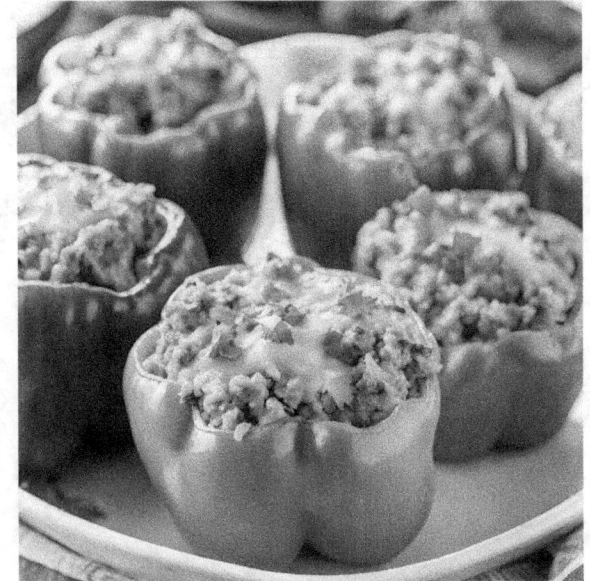

6. Spicy Chicken and Hummus Pita

Ingredients:
- 2 boneless, skinless chicken breasts, cut into strips
- 1 tablespoon olive oil
- 1 teaspoon paprika
- 1/2 teaspoon cumin
- 1/4 teaspoon cayenne pepper
- 1/2 cup hummus
- 1/2 cucumber, sliced
- 1/2 red onion, thinly sliced
- 4 whole wheat pita breads
- 1/4 cup chopped fresh parsley

Instructions:
1. In a medium bowl, combine the chicken strips, olive oil, paprika, cumin, and cayenne pepper. Mix well to coat the chicken.
2. Heat a large skillet over medium-high heat. Add the chicken strips and cook until fully cooked and browned, about 5-7 minutes.
3. Warm the pita breads in a skillet or microwave.
4. Spread a layer of hummus on each pita bread.
5. Top with the cooked chicken strips, cucumber slices, red onion slices, and chopped parsley.
6. Serve immediately.

Nutrition Info per Serving:
- Calories: 350
- Protein: 25g
- Carbohydrates: 35g
- Fat: 12g
- Fiber: 7g

Servings:
- Serves 4

Cooking Time:
- **Total: 20 minutes**

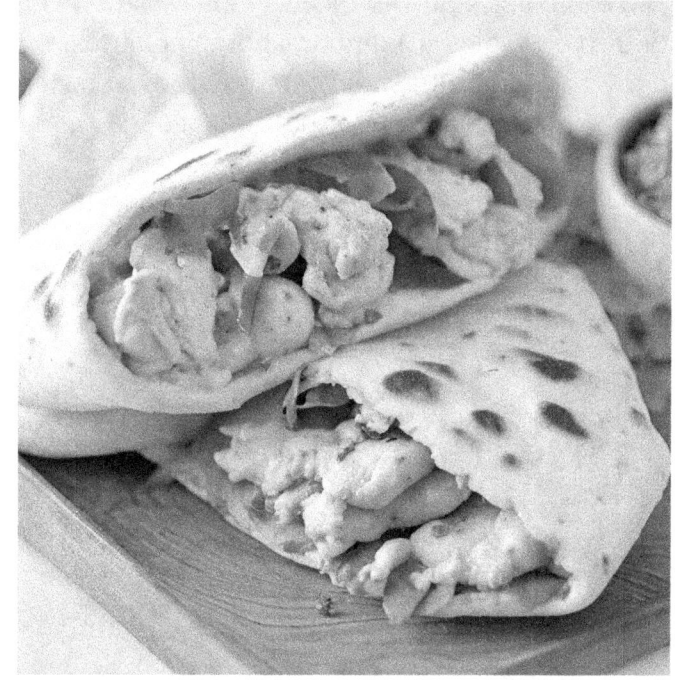

7. Turkey Meatball Soup

Ingredients:
- 1 pound ground turkey
- 1/4 cup breadcrumbs
- 1/4 cup grated Parmesan cheese
- 1 large egg
- 1 teaspoon garlic powder
- 1 teaspoon dried oregano
- 1 tablespoon olive oil
- 1 small onion, diced
- 2 carrots, sliced
- 2 celery stalks, sliced
- 2 cloves garlic, minced
- 6 cups low-sodium chicken broth
- 1 cup diced tomatoes
- 1 cup spinach leaves, chopped
- 1 teaspoon dried basil

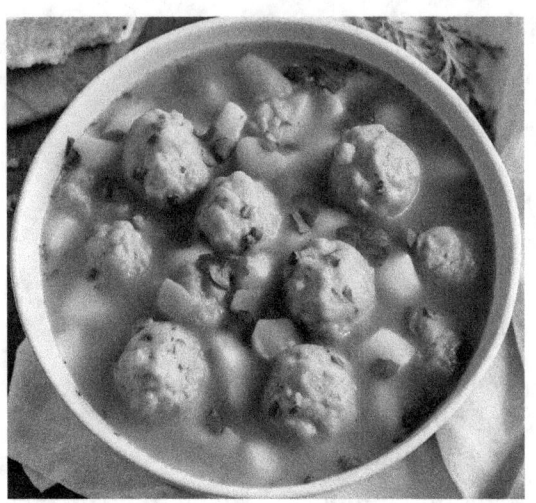

Instructions:
1. In a large bowl, combine the ground turkey, breadcrumbs, Parmesan cheese, egg, garlic powder, and oregano. Mix well and form into small meatballs.
2. Heat the olive oil in a large pot over medium heat. Add the meatballs and cook until browned on all sides, about 5-7 minutes. Remove from the pot and set aside.
3. In the same pot, add the diced onion, carrots, celery, and minced garlic. Cook until the vegetables are tender, about 5 minutes.
4. Add the chicken broth and diced tomatoes to the pot. Bring to a boil.
5. Return the meatballs to the pot and reduce the heat to a simmer. Cook for 15 minutes, until the meatballs are fully cooked.
6. Stir in the chopped spinach and dried basil. Cook for an additional 2-3 minutes until the spinach is wilted.
7. Serve immediately.

Nutrition Info per Serving:
- Calories: 250
- Protein: 25g
- Carbohydrates: 18g
- Fat: 10g
- Fiber: 3g

Servings:
- Serves 6

Cooking Time:
- Total: 35 minutes

8. Cajun Chicken Quinoa Bowl

Ingredients:
- 2 boneless, skinless chicken breasts
- 1 tablespoon olive oil
- 1 teaspoon Cajun seasoning
- 1 cup quinoa, rinsed
- 2 cups low-sodium chicken broth
- 1 red bell pepper, diced
- 1 cup cherry tomatoes, halved
- 1/2 cup corn kernels (fresh or frozen)
- 1/4 cup chopped green onions
- 1/4 cup chopped fresh cilantro

Instructions:
1. Rub the chicken breasts with olive oil and Cajun seasoning.
2. Heat a large skillet over medium heat. Add the chicken breasts and cook until browned and fully cooked, about 6-7 minutes per side. Remove from the skillet and let rest before slicing.
3. In a medium saucepan, bring the chicken broth to a boil. Add the quinoa, reduce the heat to low, cover, and simmer for 15 minutes until the quinoa is cooked and the liquid is absorbed.
4. In the same skillet used for the chicken, add the diced red bell pepper and cook for 3-4 minutes until slightly tender.
5. In a large bowl, combine the cooked quinoa, bell pepper, cherry tomatoes, corn, green onions, and cilantro.
6. Top with the sliced chicken.
7. Serve immediately.

Nutrition Info per Serving:
- Calories: 350
- Protein: 30g
- Carbohydrates: 35g
- Fat: 12g
- Fiber: 5g

Servings:
- Serves 4

Cooking Time:
- **Total: 30 minutes**

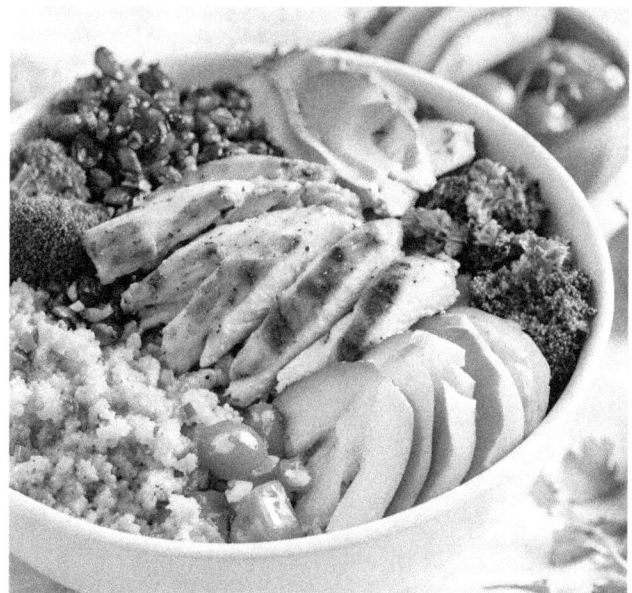

9. Balsamic Glazed Chicken Breasts

Ingredients:
- 4 boneless, skinless chicken breasts
- 2 tablespoons olive oil
- 1/4 cup balsamic vinegar
- 1/4 cup chicken broth
- 1 tablespoon honey
- 2 cloves garlic, minced
- 1 teaspoon dried rosemary

Instructions:
1. Heat the olive oil in a large skillet over medium-high heat.
2. Add the chicken breasts and cook until golden brown on both sides, about 4-5 minutes per side. Remove from the skillet and set aside.
3. In the same skillet, add the balsamic vinegar, chicken broth, honey, minced garlic, and dried rosemary. Stir to combine.
4. Bring the mixture to a simmer and cook until it thickens slightly, about 2-3 minutes.
5. Return the chicken breasts to the skillet and cook for another 5-7 minutes, basting with the glaze, until the chicken is fully cooked and the internal temperature reaches 165°F (75°C).
6. Serve immediately.

Nutrition Info per Serving:
- Calories: 240
- Protein: 28g
- Carbohydrates: 10g
- Fat: 10g
- Fiber: 0g

Servings:
- Serves 4

Cooking Time:
- Total: 20 minutes

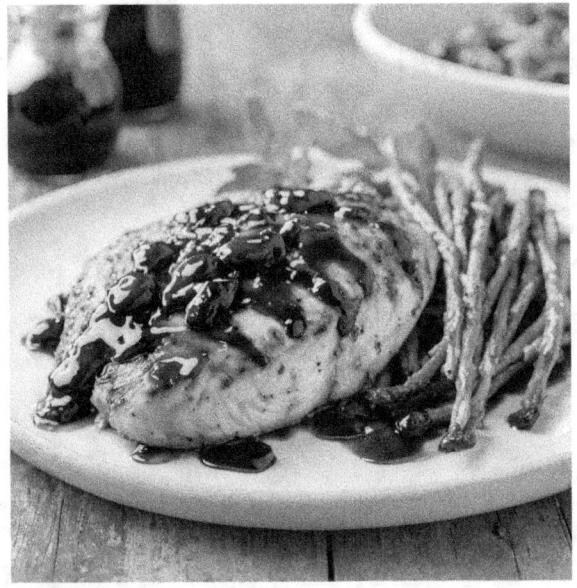

10. Chicken Ratatouille

Ingredients:
- 2 boneless, skinless chicken breasts, cut into chunks
- 2 tablespoons olive oil
- 1 small eggplant, diced
- 1 zucchini, diced
- 1 red bell pepper, diced
- 1 yellow bell pepper, diced
- 1 small onion, diced
- 2 cloves garlic, minced
- 1 can (14.5 oz) diced tomatoes
- 1 teaspoon dried basil
- 1 teaspoon dried oregano

Instructions:
1. Heat 1 tablespoon of olive oil in a large skillet over medium-high heat.
2. Add the chicken chunks and cook until browned and fully cooked, about 5-7 minutes. Remove from the skillet and set aside.
3. Add the remaining tablespoon of olive oil to the skillet.
4. Add the diced eggplant, zucchini, bell peppers, and onion. Cook until the vegetables are tender, about 7-10 minutes.
5. Stir in the minced garlic and cook for another 1-2 minutes.
6. Add the diced tomatoes, dried basil, and dried oregano. Bring to a simmer and cook for 10 minutes.
7. Return the chicken to the skillet and cook for another 5 minutes, until everything is heated through.
8. Serve immediately.

Nutrition Info per Serving:
- Calories: 280
- Protein: 26g
- Carbohydrates: 18g
- Fat: 12g
- Fiber: 6g

Servings:
- Serves 4

Cooking Time:
- **Total: 30 minutes**

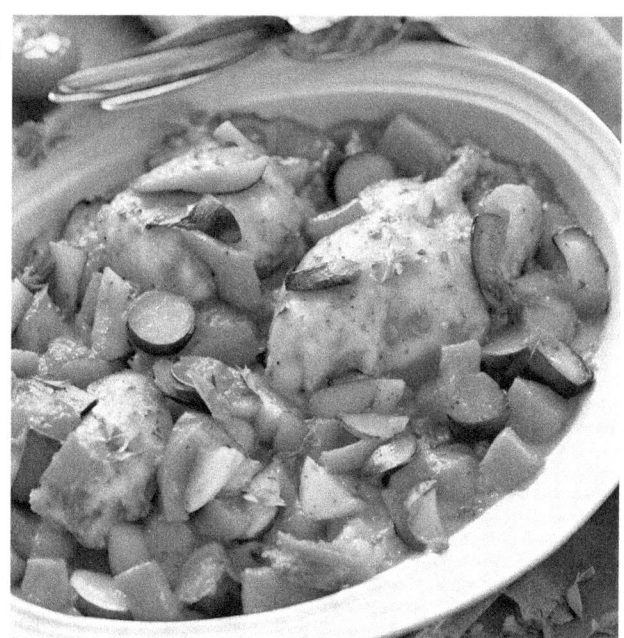

11. Mushroom and Spinach Stuffed Chicken

Ingredients:
- 4 boneless, skinless chicken breasts
- 1 tablespoon olive oil
- 1 cup mushrooms, finely chopped
- 1 cup fresh spinach, chopped
- 1/4 cup grated Parmesan cheese
- 2 cloves garlic, minced
- 1 teaspoon dried thyme

Instructions:
1. Preheat the oven to 375°F (190°C).
2. In a medium skillet, heat the olive oil over medium heat.
3. Add the mushrooms and garlic, cooking until the mushrooms are tender, about 5 minutes.
4. Stir in the chopped spinach and cook until wilted, about 2 minutes.
5. Remove from heat and stir in the grated Parmesan cheese and dried thyme.
6. Using a sharp knife, carefully cut a pocket into each chicken breast.
7. Stuff each chicken breast with the mushroom and spinach mixture.
8. Place the stuffed chicken breasts in a baking dish.
9. Bake for 25-30 minutes, or until the chicken is fully cooked and reaches an internal temperature of 165°F (75°C).
10. Serve immediately.

Nutrition Info per Serving:
- Calories: 300
- Protein: 34g
- Carbohydrates: 5g
- Fat: 15g
- Fiber: 2g

Servings:
- Serves 4

Cooking Time:
- **Total: 35 minutes**

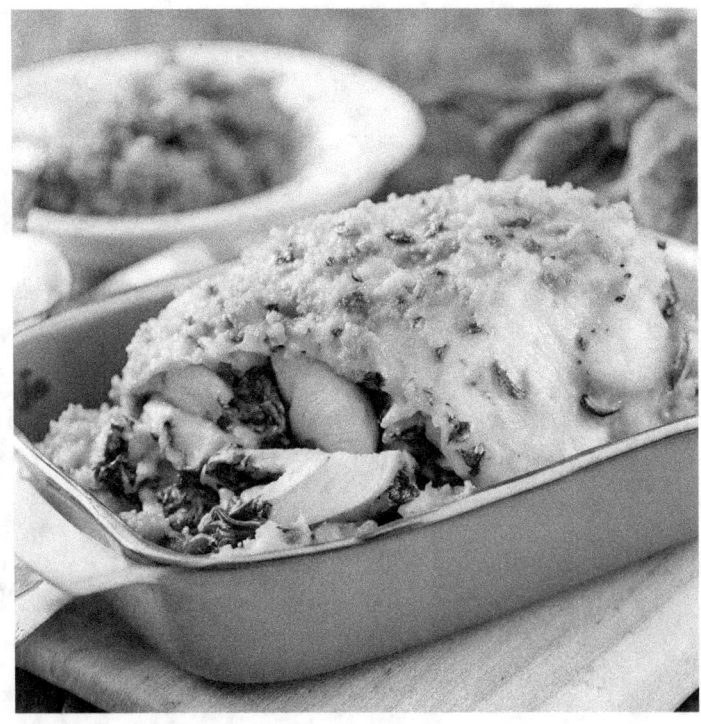

12. Chicken and Broccoli Alfredo

Ingredients:
- 2 boneless, skinless chicken breasts, cut into strips
- 2 tablespoons olive oil
- 2 cups broccoli florets
- 2 cloves garlic, minced
- 1 cup low-fat milk
- 1/2 cup grated Parmesan cheese
- 1/4 cup low-fat cream cheese
- 1/2 teaspoon dried basil
- 1/2 teaspoon dried oregano
- 8 oz whole wheat fettuccine

Instructions:
1. Cook the whole wheat fettuccine according to package instructions. Drain and set aside.
2. In a large skillet, heat 1 tablespoon of olive oil over medium heat.
3. Add the chicken strips and cook until browned and fully cooked, about 5-7 minutes. Remove from the skillet and set aside.
4. Add the remaining tablespoon of olive oil to the skillet.
5. Add the broccoli florets and cook until tender, about 5 minutes.
6. Stir in the minced garlic and cook for another 1-2 minutes.
7. Reduce the heat to low and add the low-fat milk, Parmesan cheese, and cream cheese. Stir until the cheese is melted and the sauce is smooth.
8. Stir in the dried basil and oregano.
9. Return the chicken to the skillet and stir to combine.
10. Add the cooked fettuccine to the skillet and toss to coat with the sauce.
11. Serve immediately.

Nutrition Info per Serving:
- Calories: 400
- Protein: 28g
- Carbohydrates: 45g
- Fat: 15g
- Fiber: 8g

Servings:
- Serves 4

Cooking Time:
- Total: 30 minutes

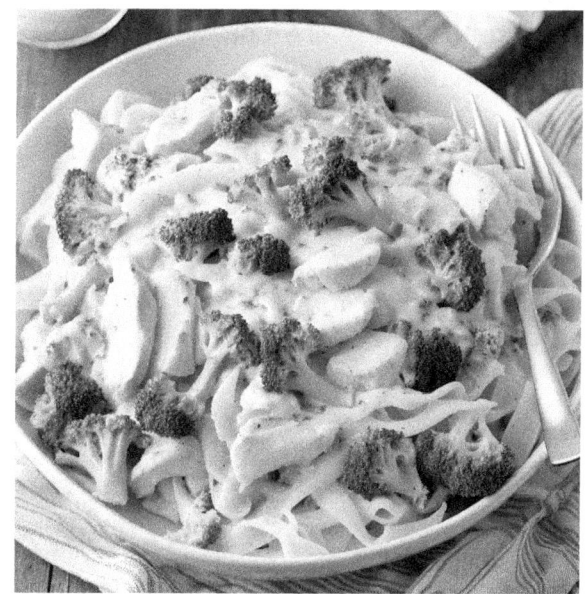

13. Curried Chicken Salad

Ingredients:
- 2 boneless, skinless chicken breasts, cooked and shredded
- 1/2 cup plain Greek yogurt
- 1/4 cup mayonnaise
- 1 tablespoon curry powder
- 1/4 cup diced celery
- 1/4 cup chopped apple
- 1/4 cup chopped pecans
- 1/4 cup raisins

Instructions:
1. In a large bowl, combine the Greek yogurt, mayonnaise, and curry powder. Mix well.
2. Add the shredded chicken, diced celery, chopped apple, chopped pecans, and raisins to the bowl.
3. Stir until all ingredients are well combined and evenly coated with the curry dressing.
4. Serve immediately or refrigerate until ready to eat.

Nutrition Info per Serving:
- Calories: 250
- Protein: 20g
- Carbohydrates: 15g
- Fat: 12g
- Fiber: 2g

Servings:
- Serves 4

Cooking Time:
- Total: 15 minutes (using pre-cooked chicken)

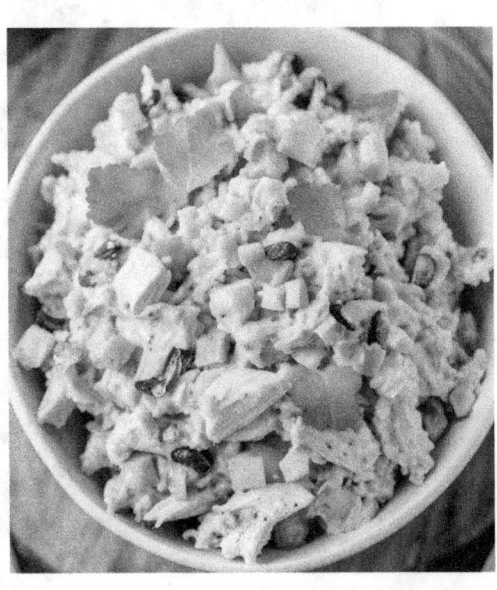

14. Garlic and Herb Roasted Turkey Breast

Ingredients:
- 1 boneless turkey breast (about 2 pounds)
- 2 tablespoons olive oil
- 4 cloves garlic, minced
- 1 tablespoon dried rosemary
- 1 tablespoon dried thyme
- 1 tablespoon lemon juice

Instructions:
1. Preheat the oven to 375°F (190°C).
2. In a small bowl, combine the olive oil, minced garlic, dried rosemary, dried thyme, and lemon juice.
3. Rub the garlic and herb mixture all over the turkey breast.
4. Place the turkey breast in a roasting pan.
5. Roast for 45-55 minutes, or until the internal temperature reaches 165°F (75°C).
6. Let the turkey rest for 10 minutes before slicing and serving.

Nutrition Info per Serving:
- Calories: 220
- Protein: 35g
- Carbohydrates: 2g
- Fat: 8g
- Fiber: 0g

Servings:
- Serves 6

Cooking Time:
- **Total: 65 minutes**

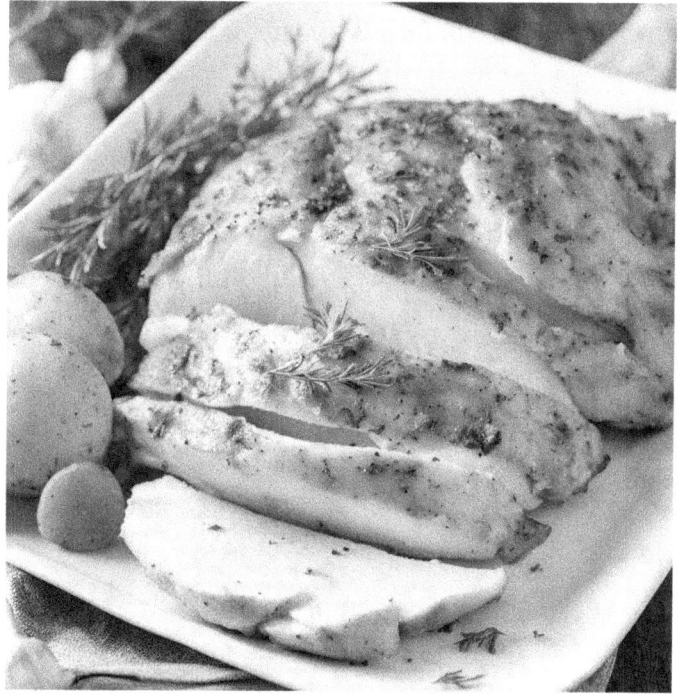

15. Turkey and Sweet Potato Skillet

Ingredients:
- 1 pound ground turkey
- 2 tablespoons olive oil
- 1 large sweet potato, peeled and diced
- 1 small onion, diced
- 2 cloves garlic, minced
- 1 teaspoon ground cumin
- 1/2 teaspoon smoked paprika
- 1/4 teaspoon red pepper flakes (optional)
- 1/2 cup chicken broth
- 2 cups fresh spinach, chopped

Instructions:
1. Heat 1 tablespoon of olive oil in a large skillet over medium heat.
2. Add the diced sweet potato and cook until slightly tender, about 5-7 minutes. Remove from the skillet and set aside.
3. Add the remaining tablespoon of olive oil to the skillet.
4. Add the diced onion and cook until translucent, about 3-4 minutes.
5. Add the minced garlic, ground cumin, smoked paprika, and red pepper flakes (if using). Cook for another minute until fragrant.
6. Add the ground turkey and cook until browned and fully cooked, about 5-7 minutes.
7. Return the sweet potatoes to the skillet and add the chicken broth. Cook until the sweet potatoes are fully tender and the liquid has mostly evaporated, about 5 minutes.
8. Stir in the chopped spinach and cook until wilted, about 2 minutes.
9. Serve immediately.

Nutrition Info per Serving:
- Calories: 300
- Protein: 25g
- Carbohydrates: 25g
- Fat: 12g
- Fiber: 5g

Servings:
- Serves 4

Cooking Time:
- Total: 25 minutes

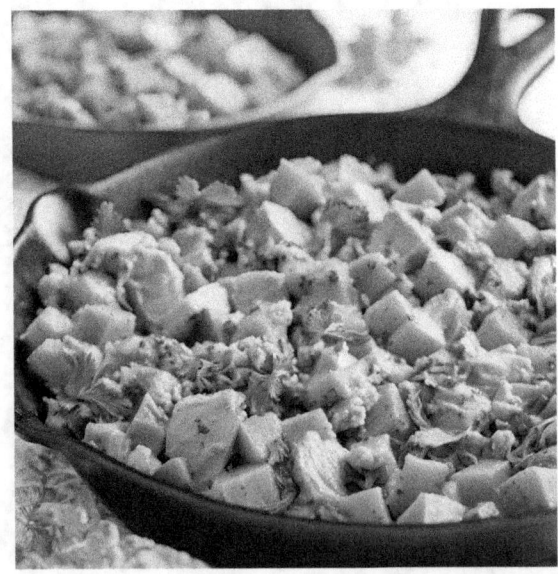

16. Buffalo Chicken Stuffed Zucchini Boats

Ingredients:
- 4 medium zucchinis, halved lengthwise and seeds removed
- 2 boneless, skinless chicken breasts, cooked and shredded
- 1/2 cup buffalo sauce
- 1/4 cup plain Greek yogurt
- 1/2 cup shredded cheddar cheese
- 2 tablespoons chopped green onions

Instructions:
1. Preheat the oven to 375°F (190°C).
2. In a medium bowl, combine the shredded chicken, buffalo sauce, and Greek yogurt. Mix well.
3. Place the zucchini halves in a baking dish.
4. Spoon the buffalo chicken mixture into each zucchini half.
5. Sprinkle the shredded cheddar cheese on top.
6. Bake for 20-25 minutes, until the zucchinis are tender and the cheese is melted and bubbly.
7. Garnish with chopped green onions before serving.

Nutrition Info per Serving:
- Calories: 250
- Protein: 25g
- Carbohydrates: 10g
- Fat: 12g
- Fiber: 3g

Servings:
- Serves 4

Cooking Time:
- **Total: 30 minutes**

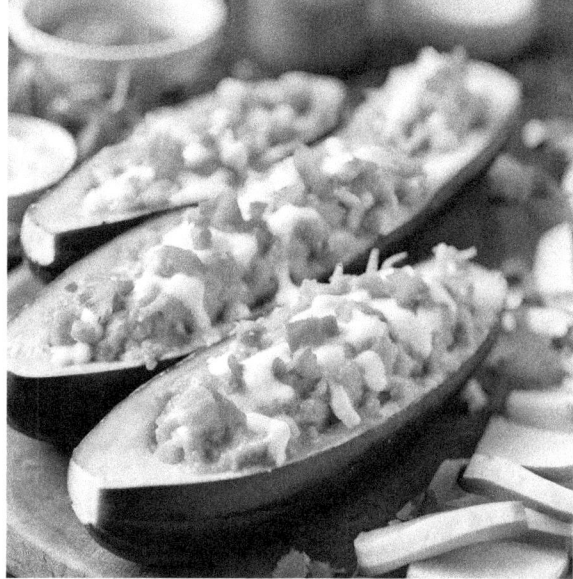

17. Pesto Chicken Wraps

Ingredients:
- 2 boneless, skinless chicken breasts, cooked and sliced
- 4 whole wheat tortillas
- 1/2 cup prepared pesto sauce
- 1 cup baby spinach leaves
- 1/2 cup shredded mozzarella cheese
- 1/4 cup sun-dried tomatoes, chopped

Instructions:
1. Warm the whole wheat tortillas in a skillet or microwave.
2. Spread 2 tablespoons of pesto sauce on each tortilla.
3. Layer the sliced chicken, baby spinach leaves, shredded mozzarella cheese, and chopped sun-dried tomatoes on each tortilla.
4. Roll up the tortillas tightly to form wraps.
5. Serve immediately or refrigerate until ready to eat.

Nutrition Info per Serving:
- Calories: 350
- Protein: 28g
- Carbohydrates: 25g
- Fat: 16g
- Fiber: 5g

Servings:
- Serves 4

Cooking Time:
- **Total: 10 minutes**

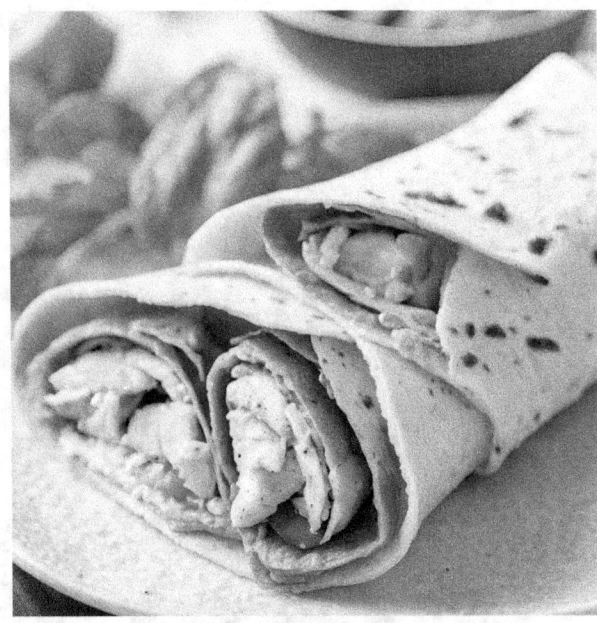

18. Herb-Roasted Chicken Thighs

Ingredients:
- 6 bone-in, skin-on chicken thighs
- 2 tablespoons olive oil
- 2 cloves garlic, minced
- 1 teaspoon dried rosemary
- 1 teaspoon dried thyme
- 1 teaspoon paprika
- 1 tablespoon lemon juice

Instructions:
1. Preheat the oven to 400°F (200°C).
2. In a small bowl, combine the olive oil, minced garlic, dried rosemary, dried thyme, paprika, and lemon juice.
3. Rub the herb mixture all over the chicken thighs, ensuring they are well coated.
4. Place the chicken thighs in a baking dish.
5. Roast for 35-40 minutes, or until the chicken is fully cooked and the internal temperature reaches 165°F (75°C).
6. Let the chicken rest for a few minutes before serving.

Nutrition Info per Serving:
- Calories: 300
- Protein: 20g
- Carbohydrates: 2g
- Fat: 24g
- Fiber: 1g

Servings:
- **Serves 6**

Cooking Time:
- **Total: 45 minutes**

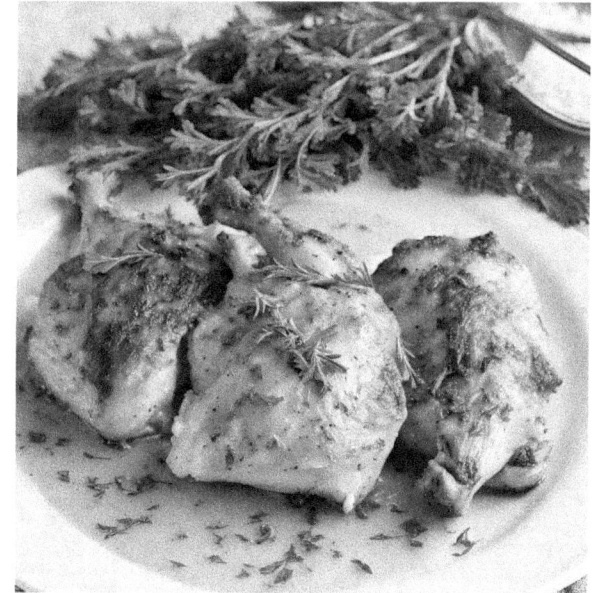

19. Lemon Garlic Turkey Burgers

Ingredients:
- 1 pound ground turkey
- 2 cloves garlic, minced
- 1 tablespoon lemon zest
- 1 tablespoon chopped fresh parsley
- 1 teaspoon dried oregano
- 1 tablespoon olive oil

Instructions:
1. In a large bowl, combine the ground turkey, minced garlic, lemon zest, chopped parsley, and dried oregano. Mix well.
2. Form the mixture into 4 patties.
3. Heat the olive oil in a large skillet over medium heat.
4. Cook the turkey patties for 5-7 minutes per side, or until fully cooked and the internal temperature reaches 165°F (75°C).
5. Serve immediately, optionally on whole wheat buns with desired toppings.

Nutrition Info per Serving:
- Calories: 220
- Protein: 25g
- Carbohydrates: 3g
- Fat: 12g
- Fiber: 1g

Servings:
- Serves 4

Cooking Time:
- Total: 20 minutes

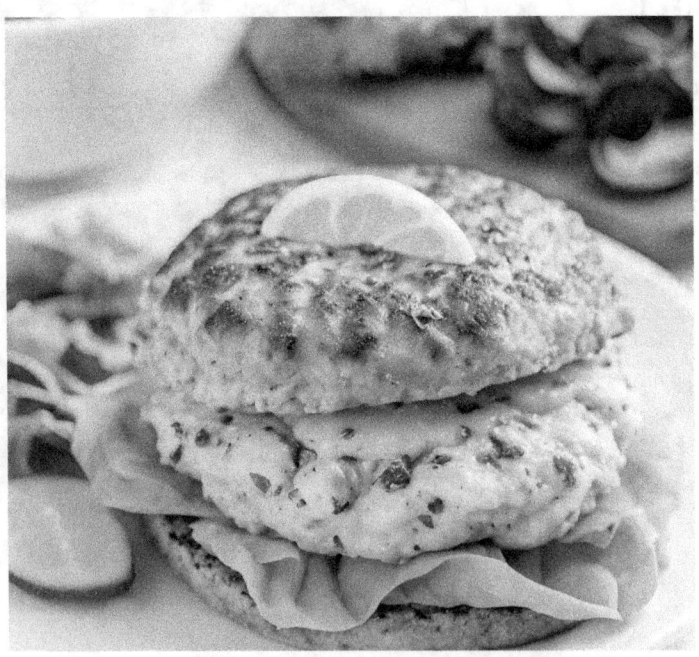

20. BBQ Turkey Meatloaf

Ingredients:
- 1 pound ground turkey
- 1/2 cup breadcrumbs
- 1/4 cup finely chopped onion
- 1/4 cup BBQ sauce (plus extra for topping)
- 1 large egg
- 1 teaspoon garlic powder
- 1 teaspoon dried thyme

Instructions:
1. Preheat the oven to 375°F (190°C).
2. In a large bowl, combine the ground turkey, breadcrumbs, chopped onion, BBQ sauce, egg, garlic powder, and dried thyme. Mix well.
3. Transfer the mixture to a loaf pan and shape it into a loaf.
4. Spread a thin layer of BBQ sauce over the top of the meatloaf.
5. Bake for 45-50 minutes, or until the meatloaf is fully cooked and the internal temperature reaches 165°F (75°C).
6. Let the meatloaf rest for 10 minutes before slicing and serving.

Nutrition Info per Serving:
- Calories: 250
- Protein: 24g
- Carbohydrates: 15g
- Fat: 10g
- Fiber: 2g

Servings:
- Serves 4

Cooking Time:
- **Total: 60 minutes**

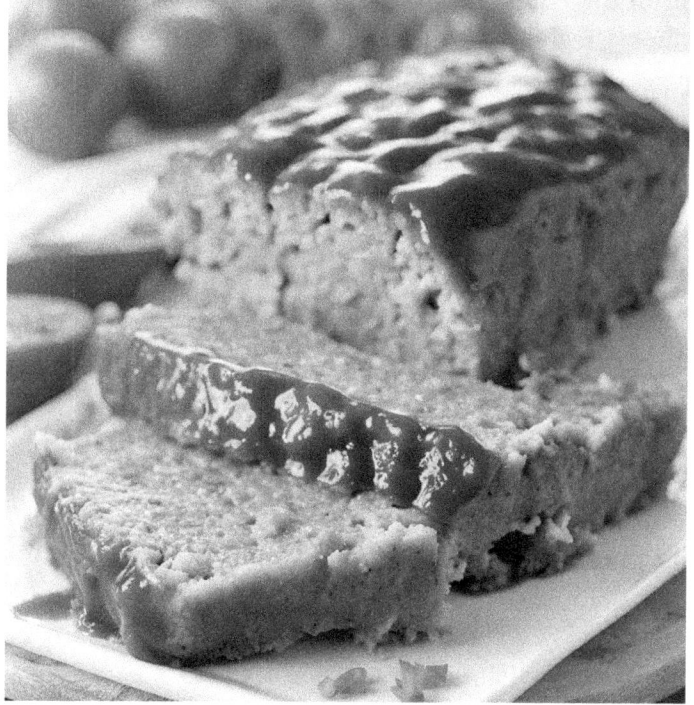

21. Chicken Vegetable Soup

Ingredients:
- 2 boneless, skinless chicken breasts, diced
- 1 tablespoon olive oil
- 1 small onion, diced
- 2 carrots, sliced
- 2 celery stalks, sliced
- 2 cloves garlic, minced
- 6 cups low-sodium chicken broth
- 1 can (14.5 oz) diced tomatoes
- 1 cup green beans, trimmed and cut into 1-inch pieces
- 1 teaspoon dried basil
- 1 teaspoon dried thyme
- 1 cup baby spinach leaves, chopped

Instructions:
1. Heat the olive oil in a large pot over medium heat.
2. Add the diced chicken and cook until browned and fully cooked, about 5-7 minutes. Remove the chicken from the pot and set aside.
3. In the same pot, add the diced onion, sliced carrots, and sliced celery. Cook until the vegetables are tender, about 5 minutes.
4. Add the minced garlic and cook for another 1-2 minutes until fragrant.
5. Pour in the chicken broth and diced tomatoes. Bring to a boil.
6. Reduce the heat to a simmer and add the green beans, dried basil, and dried thyme. Cook for 10 minutes.
7. Return the cooked chicken to the pot and stir in the chopped spinach. Cook for an additional 2-3 minutes until the spinach is wilted.
8. Serve immediately.

Nutrition Info per Serving:
- Calories: 200
- Protein: 20g
- Carbohydrates: 15g
- Fat: 7g
- Fiber: 4g

Servings:
- Serves 6

Cooking Time:
- Total: 35 minutes

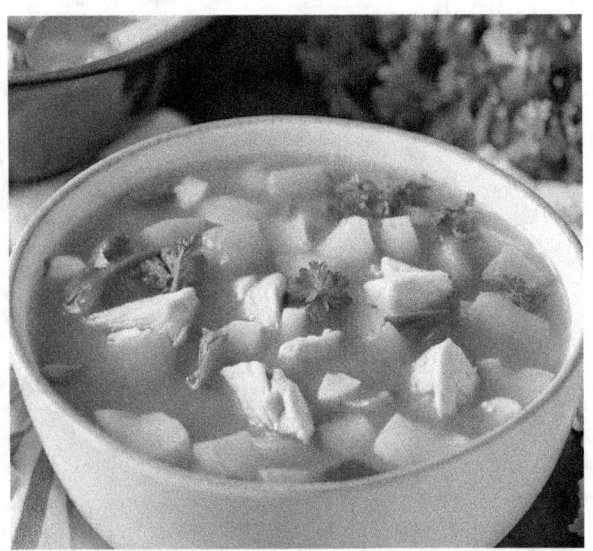

22. Asian Sesame Chicken Salad

Ingredients:
- 2 boneless, skinless chicken breasts
- 4 cups mixed salad greens
- 1 cup shredded carrots
- 1 cup thinly sliced red bell pepper
- 1/4 cup sliced green onions
- 2 tablespoons sesame seeds
- 2 tablespoons soy sauce
- 1 tablespoon rice vinegar
- 1 tablespoon sesame oil
- 1 tablespoon honey
- 1 teaspoon grated ginger
- 1 clove garlic, minced

Instructions:
1. Grill or pan-fry the chicken breasts until fully cooked, about 6-7 minutes per side. Let cool, then slice thinly.
2. In a large bowl, combine the mixed salad greens, shredded carrots, sliced red bell pepper, and sliced green onions.
3. In a small bowl, whisk together the soy sauce, rice vinegar, sesame oil, honey, grated ginger, and minced garlic to make the dressing.
4. Toss the salad with the dressing, then top with the sliced chicken and sesame seeds.
5. Serve immediately.

Nutrition Info per Serving:
- Calories: 250
- Protein: 25g
- Carbohydrates: 15g
- Fat: 10g
- Fiber: 3g

Servings:
- Serves 4

Cooking Time:
- **Total: 20 minutes**

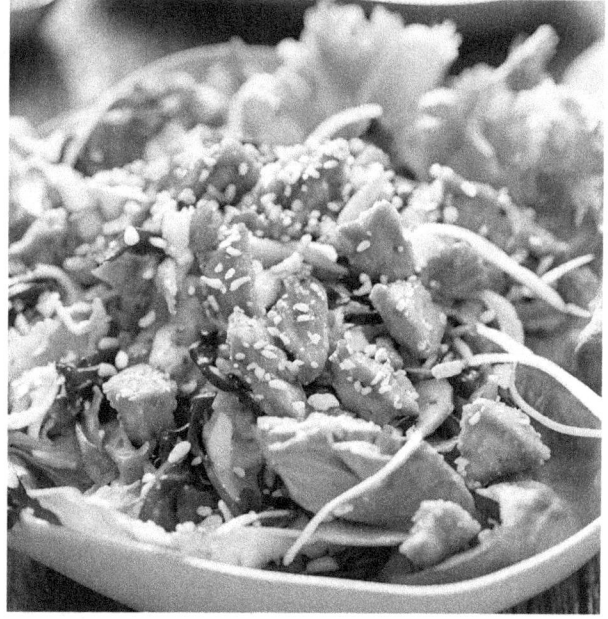

23. Chicken and Spinach Stuffed Sweet Potatoes

Ingredients:
- 4 medium sweet potatoes
- 2 boneless, skinless chicken breasts, cooked and shredded
- 1 cup fresh spinach, chopped
- 1/2 cup plain Greek yogurt
- 1/2 cup shredded mozzarella cheese
- 2 cloves garlic, minced
- 1 teaspoon dried oregano

Instructions:
1. Preheat the oven to 375°F (190°C).
2. Bake the sweet potatoes for 45-50 minutes, or until tender.
3. While the sweet potatoes are baking, mix the shredded chicken, chopped spinach, Greek yogurt, shredded mozzarella cheese, minced garlic, and dried oregano in a bowl.
4. Once the sweet potatoes are done, let them cool slightly, then cut them in half lengthwise and scoop out some of the flesh, leaving a small border.
5. Stuff the sweet potatoes with the chicken and spinach mixture.
6. Place the stuffed sweet potatoes back in the oven for an additional 10-15 minutes, until the cheese is melted and bubbly.
7. Serve immediately.

Nutrition Info per Serving:
- Calories: 350
- Protein: 25g
- Carbohydrates: 45g
- Fat: 10g
- Fiber: 7g

Servings:
- Serves 4

Cooking Time:
- Total: 65 minutes

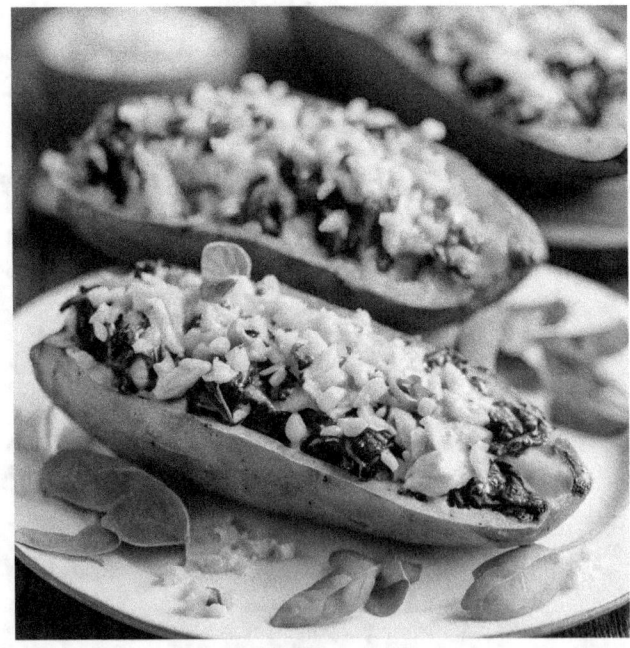

24. Turkey and Quinoa Meatballs

Ingredients:
- 1 pound ground turkey
- 1/2 cup cooked quinoa
- 1/4 cup breadcrumbs
- 1 large egg
- 2 cloves garlic, minced
- 1/4 cup grated Parmesan cheese
- 1 teaspoon dried basil
- 1 teaspoon dried oregano

Instructions:
1. Preheat the oven to 375°F (190°C).
2. In a large bowl, combine the ground turkey, cooked quinoa, breadcrumbs, egg, minced garlic, grated Parmesan cheese, dried basil, and dried oregano. Mix well.
3. Form the mixture into small meatballs and place them on a baking sheet lined with parchment paper.
4. Bake for 20-25 minutes, or until the meatballs are fully cooked and the internal temperature reaches 165°F (75°C).
5. Serve immediately.

Nutrition Info per Serving:
- Calories: 200
- Protein: 20g
- Carbohydrates: 10g
- Fat: 8g
- Fiber: 2g

Servings:
- Serves 4

Cooking Time:
- **Total: 30 minutes**

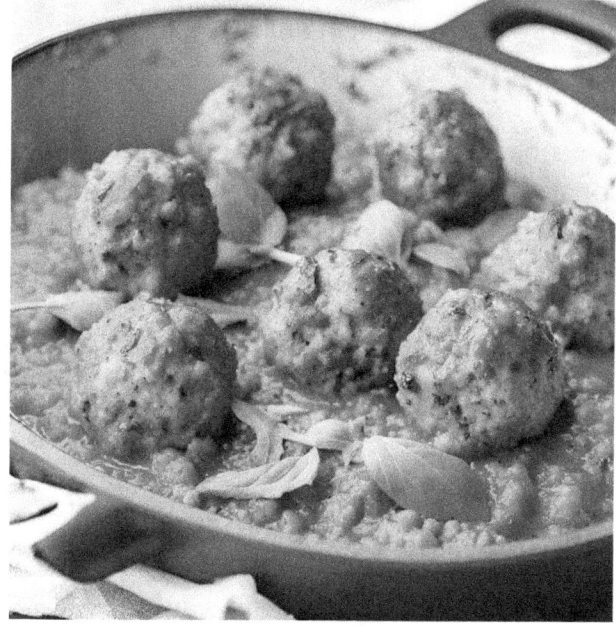

25. Chicken and Lentil Stew

Ingredients:
- 2 boneless, skinless chicken breasts, diced
- 1 tablespoon olive oil
- 1 small onion, diced
- 2 carrots, sliced
- 2 celery stalks, sliced
- 2 cloves garlic, minced
- 1 cup dried lentils, rinsed
- 6 cups low-sodium chicken broth
- 1 can (14.5 oz) diced tomatoes
- 1 teaspoon dried thyme
- 1 teaspoon dried rosemary
- 2 cups fresh spinach, chopped

Instructions:
1. Heat the olive oil in a large pot over medium heat.
2. Add the diced chicken and cook until browned and fully cooked, about 5-7 minutes. Remove the chicken from the pot and set aside.
3. In the same pot, add the diced onion, sliced carrots, and sliced celery. Cook until the vegetables are tender, about 5 minutes.
4. Add the minced garlic and cook for another 1-2 minutes until fragrant.
5. Add the dried lentils, chicken broth, diced tomatoes, dried thyme, and dried rosemary to the pot. Bring to a boil.
6. Reduce the heat to a simmer and cook for 20-25 minutes, or until the lentils are tender.
7. Return the cooked chicken to the pot and stir in the chopped spinach. Cook for an additional 2-3 minutes until the spinach is wilted.
8. Serve immediately.

Nutrition Info per Serving:
- Calories: 300
- Protein: 25g
- Carbohydrates: 35g
- Fat: 6g
- Fiber: 10g

Servings:
- Serves 6

Cooking Time:
- **Total: 40 minutes**

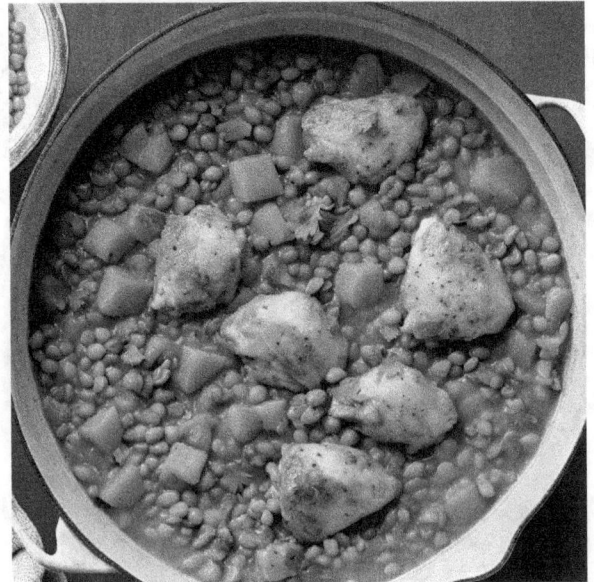

Fish and Seafood Recipes

1. Grilled Salmon with Lemon Dill Sauce

Ingredients:
- 4 salmon fillets (about 6 oz each)
- 2 tablespoons olive oil
- 2 tablespoons lemon juice
- 2 teaspoons dried dill
- 1/2 cup plain Greek yogurt
- 1 tablespoon Dijon mustard
- 1 tablespoon fresh dill, chopped
- 1 teaspoon garlic powder

Instructions:
1. Preheat the grill to medium-high heat.
2. Brush the salmon fillets with olive oil and lemon juice. Sprinkle with dried dill.
3. Grill the salmon fillets for 4-5 minutes per side, or until fully cooked and the internal temperature reaches 145°F (63°C).
4. While the salmon is grilling, prepare the lemon dill sauce. In a small bowl, mix the Greek yogurt, Dijon mustard, fresh dill, and garlic powder until well combined.
5. Serve the grilled salmon with the lemon dill sauce.

Nutrition Info per Serving:
- Calories: 350
- Protein: 30g
- Carbohydrates: 3g
- Fat: 22g
- Fiber: 0g

Servings:
- Serves 4

Cooking Time:
- **Total: 15 minutes**

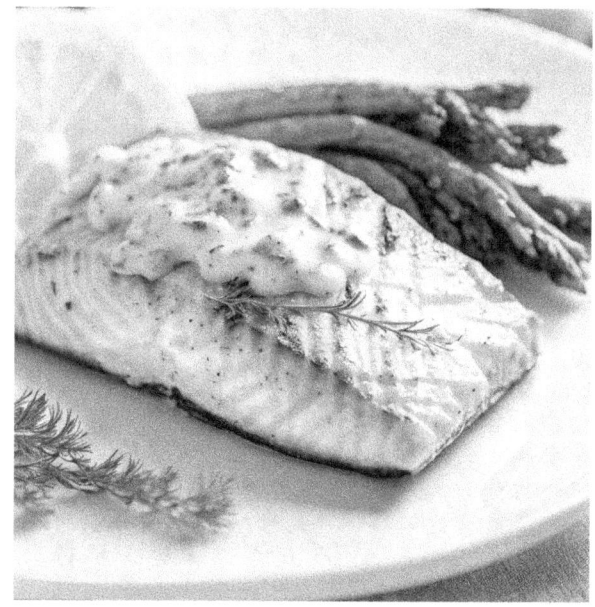

2. Shrimp and Avocado Salad

Ingredients:
- 1 pound large shrimp, peeled and deveined
- 2 tablespoons olive oil
- 2 cloves garlic, minced
- 1 tablespoon lime juice
- 1 avocado, diced
- 1 cup cherry tomatoes, halved
- 1/2 cup red onion, finely chopped
- 2 cups mixed salad greens
- 1 tablespoon chopped fresh cilantro

Instructions:
1. Heat the olive oil in a large skillet over medium heat.
2. Add the minced garlic and cook for 1 minute until fragrant.
3. Add the shrimp to the skillet and cook until pink and fully cooked, about 2-3 minutes per side. Remove from heat and let cool slightly.
4. In a large bowl, combine the cooked shrimp, diced avocado, cherry tomatoes, red onion, mixed salad greens, lime juice, and chopped cilantro.
5. Toss gently to combine and serve immediately.

Nutrition Info per Serving:
- Calories: 280
- Protein: 25g
- Carbohydrates: 10g
- Fat: 16g
- Fiber: 5g

Servings:
- Serves 4

Cooking Time:
- Total: 15 minutes

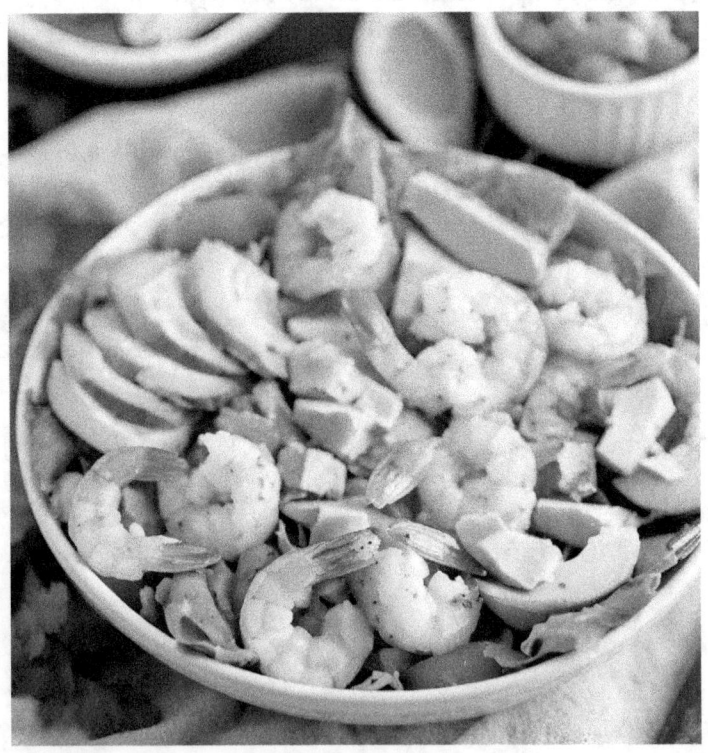

3. Baked Cod with Herb Crust

Ingredients:
- 4 cod fillets (about 6 oz each)
- 1/2 cup whole wheat breadcrumbs
- 2 tablespoons olive oil
- 1 tablespoon Dijon mustard
- 1 tablespoon lemon juice
- 1 tablespoon chopped fresh parsley
- 1 teaspoon dried thyme
- 1 teaspoon garlic powder

Instructions:
1. Preheat the oven to 375°F (190°C).
2. In a small bowl, combine the breadcrumbs, olive oil, chopped parsley, dried thyme, and garlic powder. Mix well.
3. Place the cod fillets in a baking dish.
4. Spread a thin layer of Dijon mustard over each fillet, then drizzle with lemon juice.
5. Press the breadcrumb mixture onto the top of each fillet.
6. Bake for 15-20 minutes, or until the fish is fully cooked and flakes easily with a fork.
7. Serve immediately.

Nutrition Info per Serving:
- Calories: 250
- Protein: 28g
- Carbohydrates: 12g
- Fat: 10g
- Fiber: 2g

Servings:
- Serves 4

Cooking Time:
- **Total: 25 minutes**

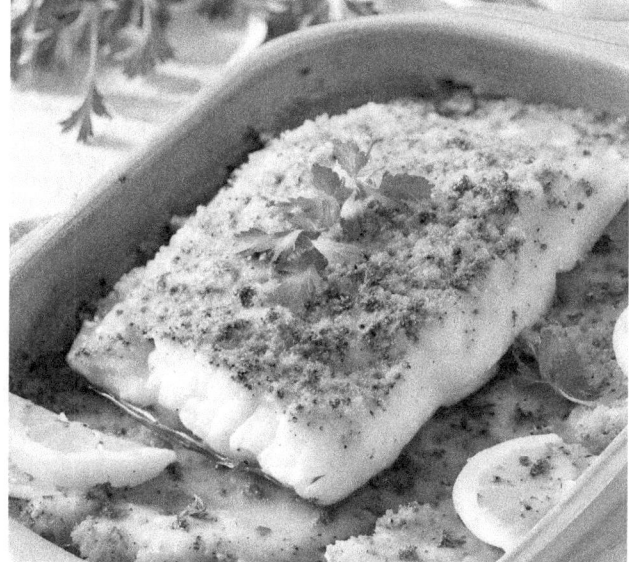

4. Tuna Nicoise Salad

Ingredients:
- 2 cans (5 oz each) tuna packed in water, drained
- 4 cups mixed salad greens
- 1 cup cherry tomatoes, halved
- 1/2 cup thinly sliced red onion
- 1/2 cup sliced black olives
- 1/2 cup green beans, blanched and cooled
- 2 hard-boiled eggs, quartered
- 1/4 cup olive oil
- 2 tablespoons lemon juice
- 1 tablespoon Dijon mustard
- 1 teaspoon dried basil
- 1 clove garlic, minced

Instructions:
1. In a small bowl, whisk together the olive oil, lemon juice, Dijon mustard, dried basil, and minced garlic to make the dressing.
2. In a large bowl, combine the mixed salad greens, cherry tomatoes, red onion, black olives, and green beans.
3. Add the drained tuna to the salad and gently toss to combine.
4. Arrange the salad on plates and top with the quartered hard-boiled eggs.
5. Drizzle the dressing over the salad before serving.

Nutrition Info per Serving:
- Calories: 320
- Protein: 25g
- Carbohydrates: 10g
- Fat: 20g
- Fiber: 4g

Servings:
- Serves 4

Cooking Time:
- **Total: 20 minutes**

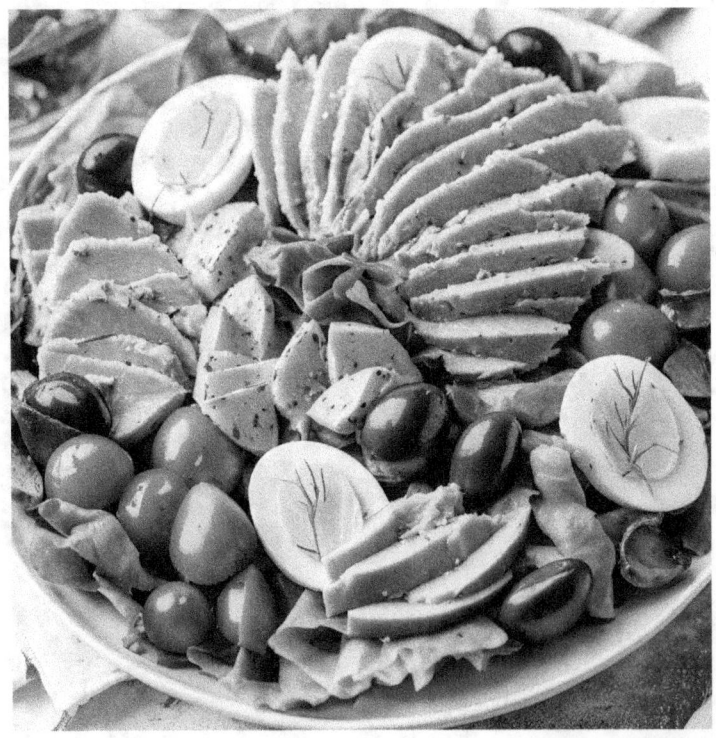

5. Seafood Paella

Ingredients:
- 1 tablespoon olive oil
- 1 onion, finely chopped
- 2 cloves garlic, minced
- 1 red bell pepper, diced
- 1 cup Arborio rice
- 1 teaspoon smoked paprika
- 1/2 teaspoon turmeric
- 1/2 cup diced tomatoes
- 4 cups low-sodium chicken broth
- 1/2 pound shrimp, peeled and deveined
- 1/2 pound mussels, cleaned
- 1/2 pound calamari rings
- 1/2 cup frozen peas
- 1/4 cup chopped fresh parsley
- 1 lemon, cut into wedges

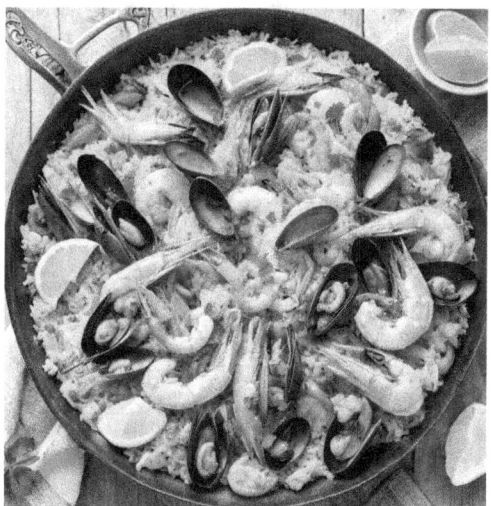

Instructions:
1. Heat the olive oil in a large skillet or paella pan over medium heat.
2. Add the chopped onion and cook until softened, about 5 minutes.
3. Stir in the minced garlic and diced red bell pepper, cooking for another 2-3 minutes.
4. Add the Arborio rice, smoked paprika, and turmeric, stirring to coat the rice with the spices.
5. Pour in the diced tomatoes and chicken broth, stirring to combine. Bring to a simmer.
6. Cook for 15 minutes, stirring occasionally, until the rice is partially cooked.
7. Add the shrimp, mussels, and calamari, tucking them into the rice. Cook for another 10 minutes, until the seafood is cooked through and the rice is tender.
8. Stir in the frozen peas and cook for an additional 2 minutes.
9. Garnish with chopped parsley and lemon wedges before serving.

Nutrition Info per Serving:
- Calories: 350
- Protein: 30g
- Carbohydrates: 45g
- Fat: 8g
- Fiber: 4g

Servings:
- Serves 4

Cooking Time:
- **Total: 40 minutes**

6. Fish Tacos with Cabbage Slaw

Ingredients:
- 1 pound white fish fillets (such as cod or tilapia)
- 2 tablespoons olive oil
- 1 teaspoon cumin
- 1 teaspoon smoked paprika
- 8 small corn tortillas
- 2 cups shredded cabbage
- 1/2 cup grated carrot
- 1/4 cup chopped fresh cilantro
- 1/4 cup plain Greek yogurt
- 1 tablespoon lime juice
- 1 teaspoon honey

Instructions:
1. Preheat the oven to 375°F (190°C).
2. Place the fish fillets on a baking sheet. Drizzle with olive oil and sprinkle with cumin and smoked paprika.
3. Bake the fish for 15-20 minutes, until fully cooked and flaky.
4. While the fish is baking, prepare the cabbage slaw. In a large bowl, combine the shredded cabbage, grated carrot, and chopped cilantro.
5. In a small bowl, mix the Greek yogurt, lime juice, and honey. Pour over the cabbage mixture and toss to combine.
6. Warm the corn tortillas in a skillet or microwave.
7. Assemble the tacos by placing pieces of baked fish on each tortilla and topping with the cabbage slaw.
8. Serve immediately.

Nutrition Info per Serving:
- Calories: 300
- Protein: 25g
- Carbohydrates: 30g
- Fat: 10g
- Fiber: 5g

Servings:
- Serves 4

Cooking Time:
- **Total: 25 minutes**

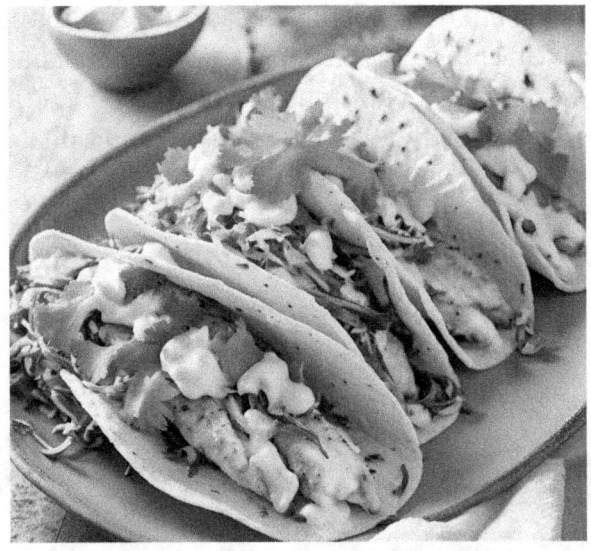

7. Grilled Mackerel with Orange Salad

Ingredients:
- 4 mackerel fillets
- 2 tablespoons olive oil
- 1 teaspoon garlic powder
- 1 teaspoon dried thyme
- 2 oranges, peeled and segmented
- 1/2 red onion, thinly sliced
- 1/4 cup chopped fresh parsley
- 1 tablespoon balsamic vinegar

Instructions:
1. Preheat the grill to medium-high heat.
2. Brush the mackerel fillets with olive oil and sprinkle with garlic powder and dried thyme.
3. Grill the mackerel fillets for 4-5 minutes per side, until fully cooked and the internal temperature reaches 145°F (63°C).
4. While the mackerel is grilling, prepare the orange salad. In a large bowl, combine the orange segments, thinly sliced red onion, and chopped parsley.
5. Drizzle the balsamic vinegar over the salad and toss to combine.
6. Serve the grilled mackerel with the orange salad on the side.

Nutrition Info per Serving:
- Calories: 350
- Protein: 30g
- Carbohydrates: 15g
- Fat: 20g
- Fiber: 3g

Servings:
- Serves 4

Cooking Time:
- **Total: 15 minutes**

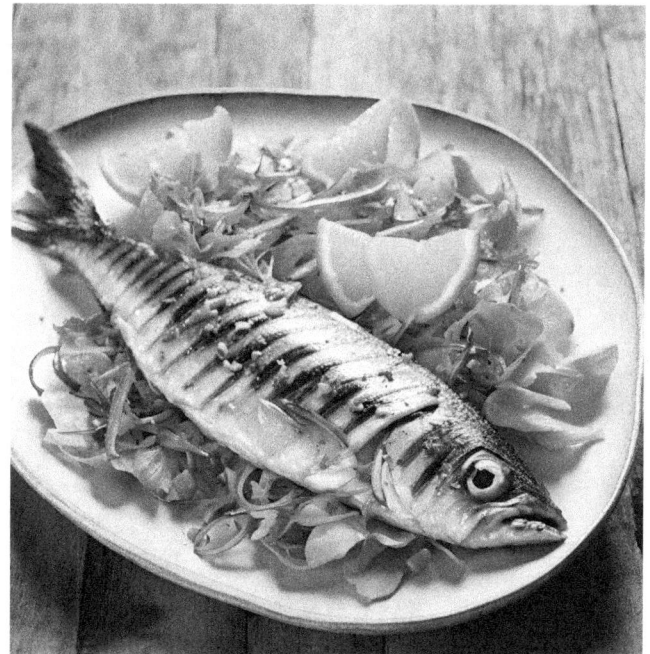

8. Smoked Salmon and Cream Cheese Omelette

Ingredients:
- 6 large eggs
- 1/4 cup milk
- 1 tablespoon olive oil
- 4 ounces smoked salmon, chopped
- 1/4 cup cream cheese, softened
- 2 tablespoons chopped fresh chives

Instructions:
1. In a medium bowl, whisk together the eggs and milk until well combined.
2. Heat the olive oil in a non-stick skillet over medium heat.
3. Pour the egg mixture into the skillet, cooking until the edges start to set, about 2-3 minutes.
4. Add the chopped smoked salmon and dollops of cream cheese to one side of the omelette.
5. Gently fold the omelette in half and cook for another 1-2 minutes, until the eggs are fully set.
6. Slide the omelette onto a plate and sprinkle with chopped fresh chives.
7. Serve immediately.

Nutrition Info per Serving:
- Calories: 300
- Protein: 22g
- Carbohydrates: 3g
- Fat: 22g
- Fiber: 0g

Servings:
- Serves 2

Cooking Time:
- **Total: 10 minutes**

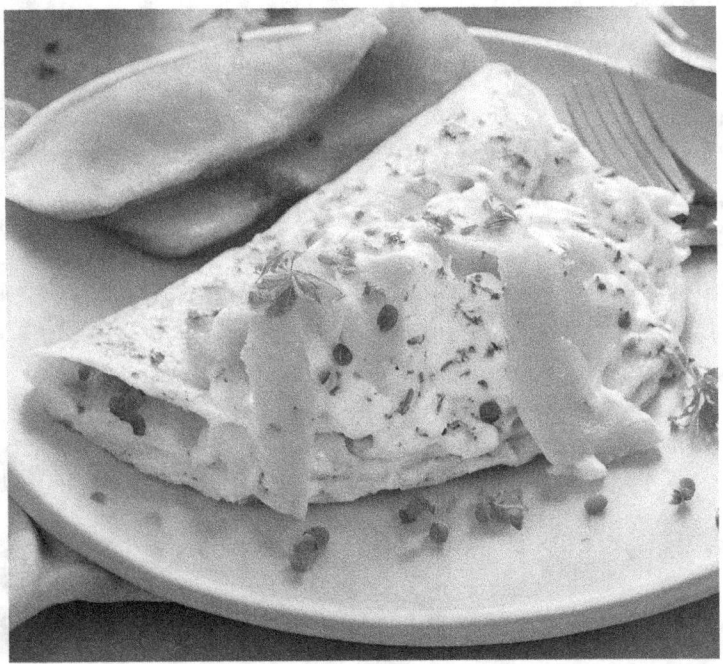

9. Scallop and Pea Risotto

Ingredients:
- 1 tablespoon olive oil
- 1 small onion, finely chopped
- 2 cloves garlic, minced
- 1 cup Arborio rice
- 1/2 cup dry white wine (optional)
- 4 cups low-sodium chicken broth, warmed
- 1 cup frozen peas
- 1 pound scallops, patted dry
- 1/4 cup grated Parmesan cheese
- 2 tablespoons chopped fresh parsley

Instructions:
1. Heat the olive oil in a large saucepan over medium heat.
2. Add the chopped onion and cook until softened, about 5 minutes.
3. Stir in the minced garlic and Arborio rice, cooking for 1-2 minutes until the rice is lightly toasted.
4. Pour in the white wine, if using, and cook until mostly absorbed.
5. Gradually add the warmed chicken broth, one ladle at a time, stirring frequently and allowing the liquid to be absorbed before adding more. Continue this process until the rice is creamy and tender, about 18-20 minutes.
6. Stir in the frozen peas and cook for an additional 2 minutes.
7. While the risotto is cooking, heat a separate skillet over medium-high heat. Sear the scallops for 2-3 minutes per side, until golden brown and cooked through.
8. Stir the grated Parmesan cheese and chopped parsley into the risotto.
9. Serve the risotto topped with the seared scallops.

Nutrition Info per Serving:
- Calories: 400
- Protein: 25g
- Carbohydrates: 45g
- Fat: 12g
- Fiber: 4g

Servings:
- Serves 4

Cooking Time:
- Total: 30 minutes

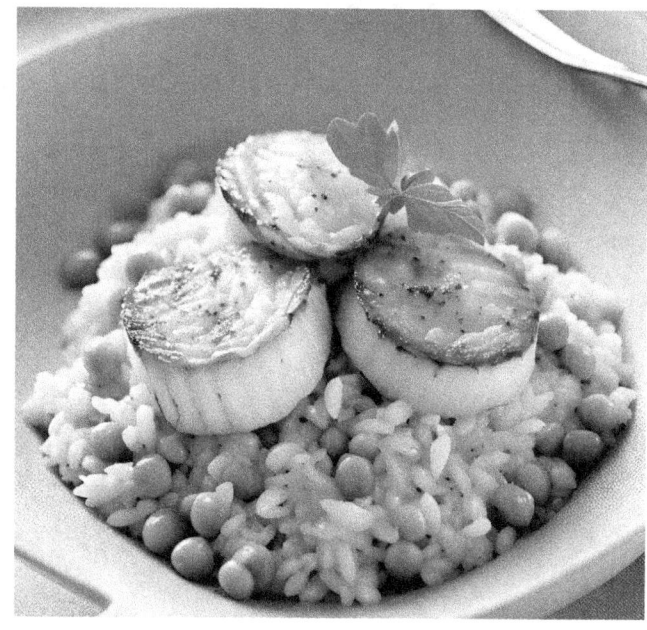

10. Mediterranean Baked Trout

Ingredients:
- 4 trout fillets
- 2 tablespoons olive oil
- 1 lemon, thinly sliced
- 1 cup cherry tomatoes, halved
- 1/2 cup Kalamata olives, pitted and sliced
- 1/4 cup red onion, thinly sliced
- 2 cloves garlic, minced
- 1 teaspoon dried oregano
- 2 tablespoons chopped fresh parsley

Instructions:
1. Preheat the oven to 375°F (190°C).
2. Place the trout fillets on a baking sheet lined with parchment paper.
3. Drizzle the fillets with olive oil and sprinkle with dried oregano.
4. Arrange the lemon slices, cherry tomatoes, Kalamata olives, red onion, and minced garlic evenly over the fillets.
5. Bake for 15-20 minutes, or until the trout is fully cooked and flakes easily with a fork.
6. Garnish with chopped fresh parsley before serving.

Nutrition Info per Serving:
- Calories: 280
- Protein: 28g
- Carbohydrates: 8g
- Fat: 16g
- Fiber: 2g

Servings:
- Serves 4

Cooking Time:
- Total: 25 minutes

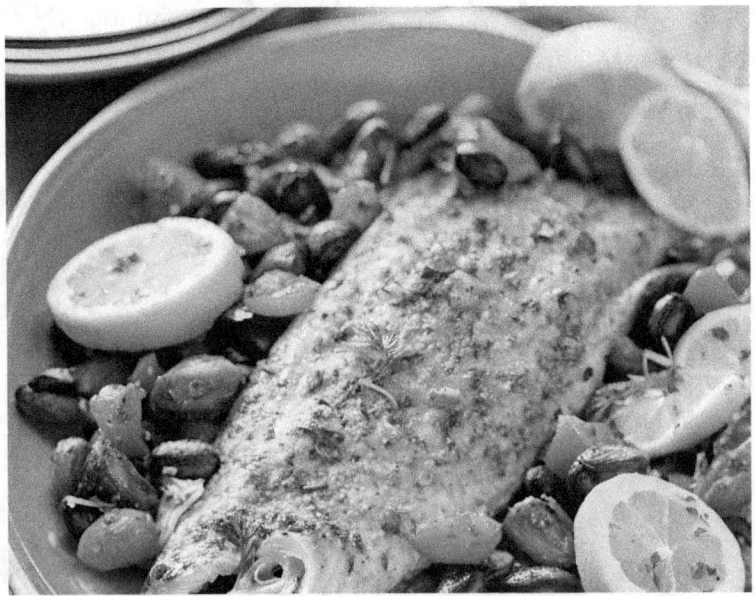

11. Pan-Seared Tilapia with Tomato Caper Sauce

Ingredients:
- 4 tilapia fillets
- 2 tablespoons olive oil
- 1 cup cherry tomatoes, halved
- 2 tablespoons capers, drained
- 2 cloves garlic, minced
- 1/4 cup fresh basil, chopped
- 1 tablespoon lemon juice

Instructions:
1. Heat 1 tablespoon of olive oil in a large skillet over medium heat.
2. Add the tilapia fillets and cook for 3-4 minutes per side, until golden brown and fully cooked. Remove from the skillet and set aside.
3. In the same skillet, add the remaining tablespoon of olive oil.
4. Add the cherry tomatoes, capers, and minced garlic. Cook for 3-4 minutes, until the tomatoes begin to soften.
5. Stir in the chopped basil and lemon juice, cooking for an additional minute.
6. Serve the tilapia fillets topped with the tomato caper sauce.

Nutrition Info per Serving:
- Calories: 250
- Protein: 30g
- Carbohydrates: 6g
- Fat: 12g
- Fiber: 2g

Servings:
- Serves 4

Cooking Time:
- **Total: 15 minutes**

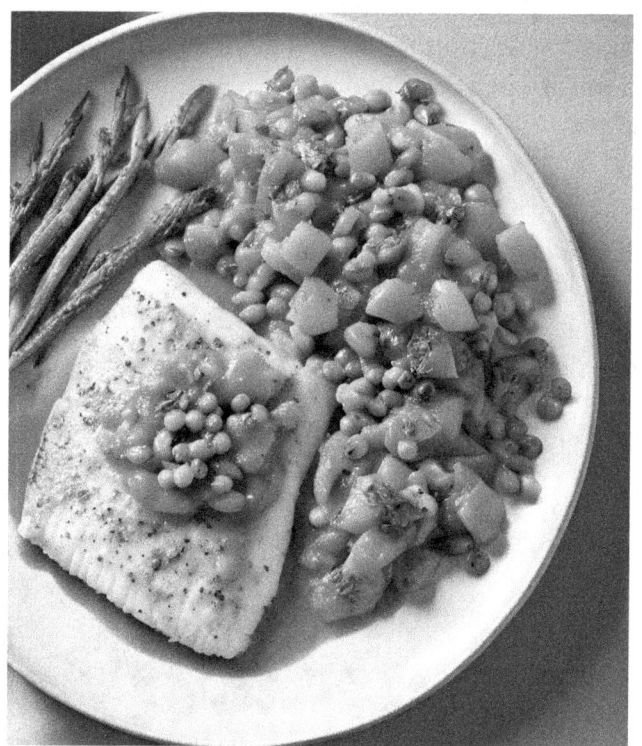

12. Spicy Shrimp Stir-Fry

Ingredients:
- 1 pound large shrimp, peeled and deveined
- 2 tablespoons olive oil
- 1 red bell pepper, sliced
- 1 yellow bell pepper, sliced
- 1 zucchini, sliced
- 2 cloves garlic, minced
- 1 tablespoon soy sauce
- 1 tablespoon sriracha sauce
- 1 teaspoon grated fresh ginger
- 1 tablespoon chopped fresh cilantro

Instructions:
1. Heat 1 tablespoon of olive oil in a large skillet or wok over medium-high heat.
2. Add the shrimp and cook until pink and fully cooked, about 2-3 minutes per side. Remove from the skillet and set aside.
3. Add the remaining tablespoon of olive oil to the skillet.
4. Add the red bell pepper, yellow bell pepper, zucchini, and minced garlic. Stir-fry for 5-7 minutes until the vegetables are tender-crisp.
5. Return the shrimp to the skillet.
6. Stir in the soy sauce, sriracha sauce, and grated ginger. Cook for another 2 minutes, until everything is heated through.
7. Garnish with chopped fresh cilantro before serving.

Nutrition Info per Serving:
- Calories: 260
- Protein: 25g
- Carbohydrates: 10g
- Fat: 12g
- Fiber: 3g

Servings:
- Serves 4

Cooking Time:
- **Total: 20 minutes**

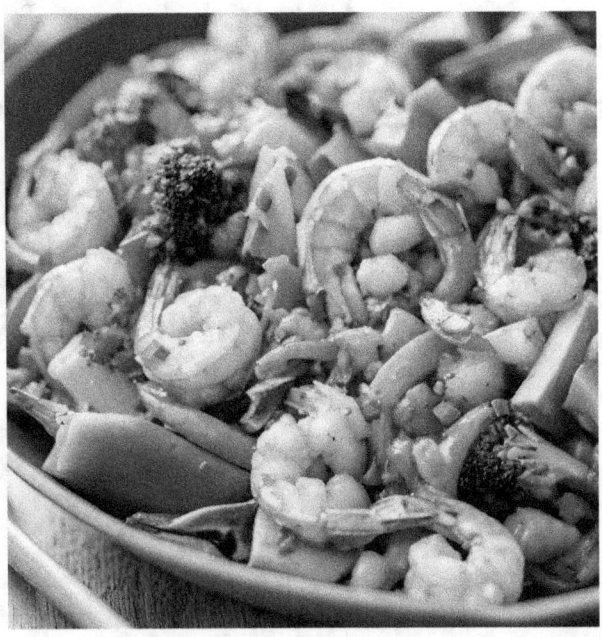

13. Salmon Quinoa Burgers

Ingredients:
- 1 pound salmon fillets, cooked and flaked
- 1 cup cooked quinoa
- 1/4 cup breadcrumbs
- 1 large egg, beaten
- 2 green onions, finely chopped
- 2 cloves garlic, minced
- 1 tablespoon lemon juice
- 1 teaspoon dried dill
- 2 tablespoons olive oil

Instructions:
1. In a large bowl, combine the flaked salmon, cooked quinoa, breadcrumbs, beaten egg, green onions, minced garlic, lemon juice, and dried dill. Mix well.
2. Form the mixture into 4 patties.
3. Heat the olive oil in a large skillet over medium heat.
4. Cook the patties for 4-5 minutes per side, until golden brown and fully cooked.
5. Serve the salmon quinoa burgers on whole wheat buns with your favorite toppings.

Nutrition Info per Serving:
- Calories: 350
- Protein: 28g
- Carbohydrates: 20g
- Fat: 18g
- Fiber: 4g

Servings:
- **Serves 4**

Cooking Time:
- **Total: 20 minutes**

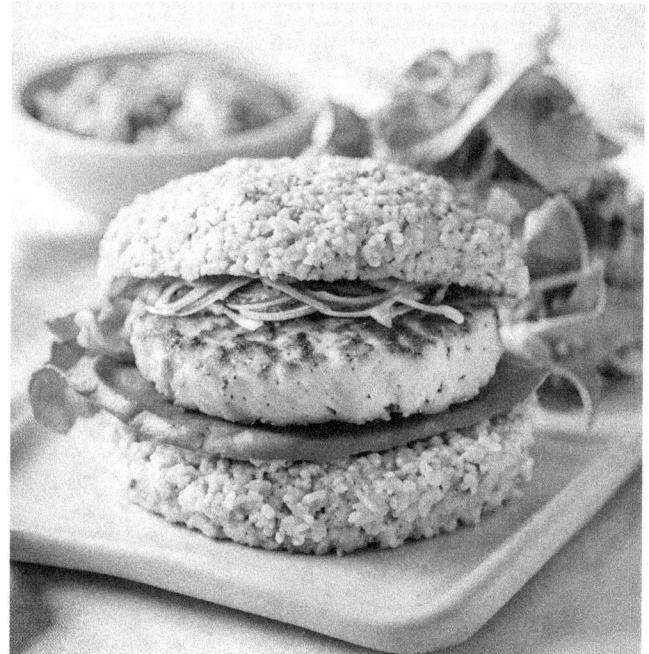

14. Fish Curry with Vegetables

Ingredients:
- 1 pound white fish fillets (such as cod or tilapia), cut into chunks
- 2 tablespoons olive oil
- 1 onion, finely chopped
- 2 cloves garlic, minced
- 1 tablespoon grated fresh ginger
- 1 tablespoon curry powder
- 1 can (14.5 oz) diced tomatoes
- 1 can (14 oz) coconut milk
- 1 cup broccoli florets
- 1 red bell pepper, sliced
- 1 zucchini, sliced
- 1/4 cup chopped fresh cilantro

Instructions:
1. Heat the olive oil in a large pot over medium heat.
2. Add the chopped onion and cook until softened, about 5 minutes.
3. Stir in the minced garlic and grated ginger, cooking for another 1-2 minutes.
4. Add the curry powder and cook for another minute until fragrant.
5. Pour in the diced tomatoes and coconut milk, stirring to combine.
6. Bring the mixture to a simmer, then add the broccoli, red bell pepper, and zucchini. Cook for 5-7 minutes until the vegetables are tender.
7. Add the fish chunks and simmer for another 5-7 minutes, until the fish is cooked through.
8. Garnish with chopped fresh cilantro before serving.

Nutrition Info per Serving:
- Calories: 320
- Protein: 25g
- Carbohydrates: 15g
- Fat: 18g
- Fiber: 4g

Servings:
- Serves 4

Cooking Time:
- Total: 30 minutes

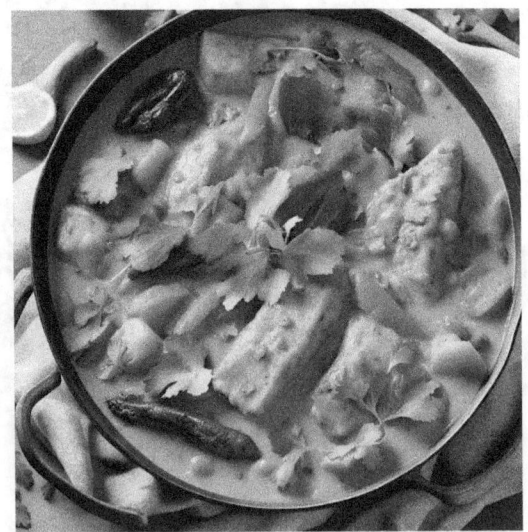

15. Pistachio-Crusted Halibut

Ingredients:
- 4 halibut fillets (about 6 oz each)
- 1/2 cup shelled pistachios, finely chopped
- 1/4 cup whole wheat breadcrumbs
- 2 tablespoons olive oil
- 1 tablespoon Dijon mustard
- 1 tablespoon lemon juice
- 1 teaspoon dried thyme

Instructions:
1. Preheat the oven to 375°F (190°C).
2. In a small bowl, combine the chopped pistachios, whole wheat breadcrumbs, and dried thyme.
3. In another small bowl, mix the olive oil, Dijon mustard, and lemon juice.
4. Brush the halibut fillets with the mustard mixture, then press the pistachio mixture onto the top of each fillet.
5. Place the fillets on a baking sheet lined with parchment paper.
6. Bake for 15-20 minutes, or until the fish is fully cooked and flakes easily with a fork.
7. Serve immediately.

Nutrition Info per Serving:
- Calories: 350
- Protein: 30g
- Carbohydrates: 10g
- Fat: 20g
- Fiber: 3g

Servings:
- Serves 4

Cooking Time:
- **Total: 25 minutes**

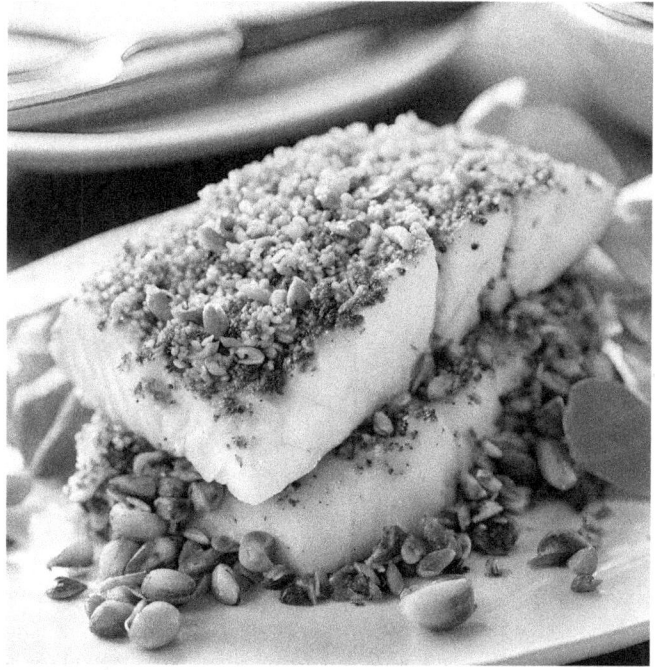

16. Oyster Mushroom and Shrimp Ramen

Ingredients:
- 1 pound large shrimp, peeled and deveined
- 2 tablespoons olive oil
- 2 cloves garlic, minced
- 1 tablespoon grated fresh ginger
- 4 cups low-sodium chicken broth
- 1 cup sliced oyster mushrooms
- 2 cups baby spinach
- 3 tablespoons soy sauce
- 2 tablespoons miso paste
- 8 oz ramen noodles
- 2 green onions, sliced
- 1 tablespoon sesame seeds

Instructions:
1. Heat the olive oil in a large pot over medium heat.
2. Add the minced garlic and grated ginger, cooking for 1-2 minutes until fragrant.
3. Pour in the chicken broth and bring to a boil.
4. Add the sliced oyster mushrooms and cook for 5 minutes.
5. Stir in the soy sauce and miso paste until well combined.
6. Add the shrimp and ramen noodles to the pot, cooking for 3-4 minutes until the shrimp are pink and the noodles are tender.
7. Stir in the baby spinach and cook for an additional 2 minutes until wilted.
8. Serve the ramen topped with sliced green onions and sesame seeds.

Nutrition Info per Serving:
- Calories: 350
- Protein: 25g
- Carbohydrates: 40g
- Fat: 10g
- Fiber: 4g

Servings:
- Serves 4

Cooking Time:
- **Total: 20 minutes**

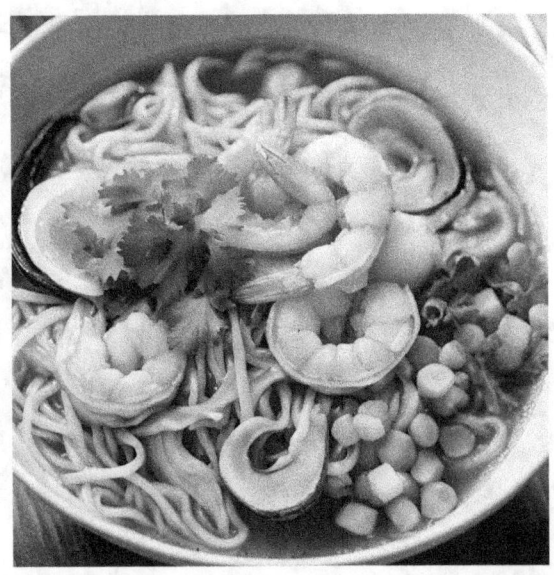

17. Thai Coconut Fish Soup

Ingredients:
- 1 pound white fish fillets (such as cod or tilapia), cut into chunks
- 2 tablespoons olive oil
- 1 onion, finely chopped
- 2 cloves garlic, minced
- 1 tablespoon grated fresh ginger
- 1 tablespoon red curry paste
- 1 can (14 oz) coconut milk
- 4 cups low-sodium chicken broth
- 1 red bell pepper, sliced
- 1 cup sliced mushrooms
- 2 tablespoons fish sauce
- 1 tablespoon lime juice
- 1/4 cup chopped fresh cilantro

Instructions:
1. Heat the olive oil in a large pot over medium heat.
2. Add the chopped onion and cook until softened, about 5 minutes.
3. Stir in the minced garlic, grated ginger, and red curry paste, cooking for another 1-2 minutes.
4. Pour in the coconut milk and chicken broth, stirring to combine.
5. Bring the mixture to a simmer, then add the red bell pepper and mushrooms. Cook for 5 minutes.
6. Add the fish chunks and simmer for another 5-7 minutes, until the fish is cooked through.
7. Stir in the fish sauce and lime juice.
8. Garnish with chopped fresh cilantro before serving.

Nutrition Info per Serving:
- Calories: 320
- Protein: 25g
- Carbohydrates: 15g
- Fat: 18g
- Fiber: 3g

Servings:
- Serves 4

Cooking Time:
- Total: 30 minutes

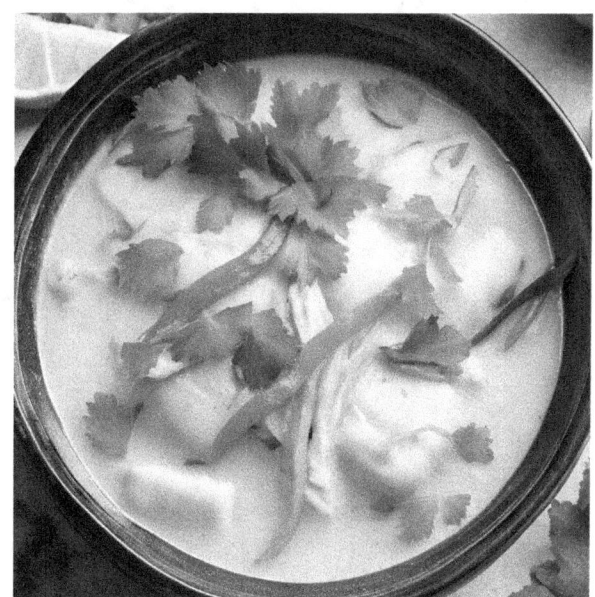

18. Sesame Seared Tuna

Ingredients:
- 4 tuna steaks (about 6 oz each)
- 2 tablespoons olive oil
- 1/4 cup sesame seeds
- 1 tablespoon soy sauce
- 1 tablespoon lemon juice
- 1 teaspoon grated fresh ginger
- 1 tablespoon chopped fresh chives

Instructions:
1. In a small bowl, combine the soy sauce, lemon juice, and grated ginger.
2. Brush the tuna steaks with the soy sauce mixture.
3. Press the sesame seeds onto both sides of each tuna steak.
4. Heat the olive oil in a large skillet over medium-high heat.
5. Sear the tuna steaks for 1-2 minutes per side, until the sesame seeds are golden brown and the tuna is cooked to your desired level of doneness.
6. Remove from heat and let rest for a few minutes.
7. Garnish with chopped fresh chives before serving.

Nutrition Info per Serving:
- Calories: 350
- Protein: 35g
- Carbohydrates: 5g
- Fat: 20g
- Fiber: 2g

Servings:
- **Serves 4**

Cooking Time:
- **Total: 15 minutes**

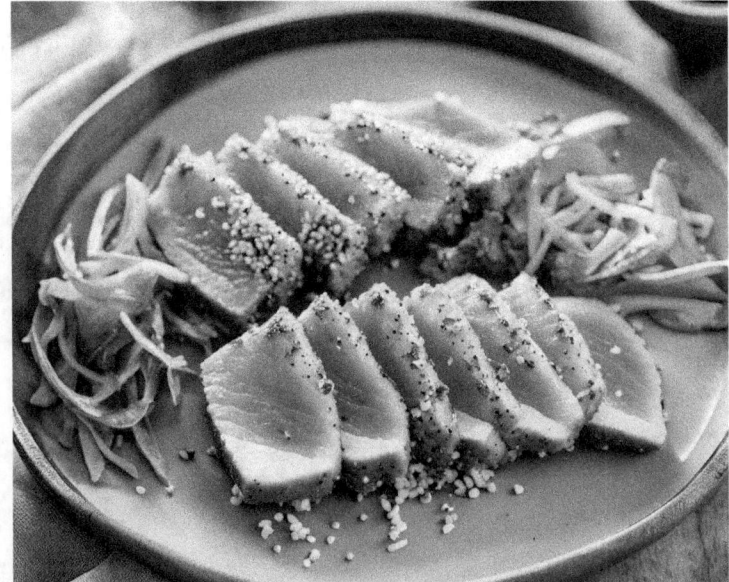

19. Garlic Butter Scallops

Ingredients:
- 1 pound sea scallops
- 2 tablespoons olive oil
- 3 tablespoons unsalted butter
- 3 cloves garlic, minced
- 1 tablespoon lemon juice
- 1 tablespoon chopped fresh parsley

Instructions:
1. Pat the scallops dry with paper towels.
2. Heat the olive oil in a large skillet over medium-high heat.
3. Add the scallops to the skillet and cook for 2-3 minutes per side, until golden brown and cooked through. Remove from the skillet and set aside.
4. In the same skillet, melt the butter over medium heat.
5. Add the minced garlic and cook for 1 minute until fragrant.
6. Stir in the lemon juice and cook for another minute.
7. Return the scallops to the skillet, tossing to coat in the garlic butter sauce.
8. Garnish with chopped fresh parsley before serving.

Nutrition Info per Serving:
- Calories: 280
- Protein: 24g
- Carbohydrates: 3g
- Fat: 18g
- Fiber: 0g

Servings:
- **Serves 4**

Cooking Time:
- **Total: 15 minutes**

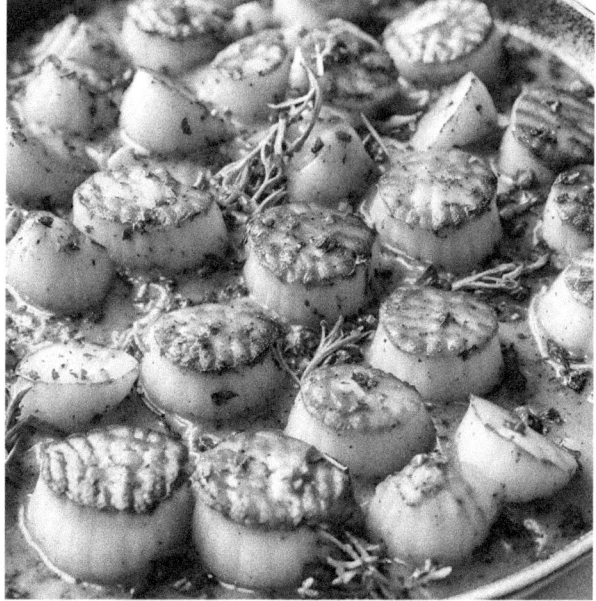

20. Grilled Shrimp and Pineapple Skewers

Ingredients:
- 1 pound large shrimp, peeled and deveined
- 2 cups fresh pineapple chunks
- 2 tablespoons olive oil
- 2 tablespoons soy sauce
- 1 tablespoon honey
- 1 teaspoon grated fresh ginger

Instructions:
1. Preheat the grill to medium-high heat.
2. In a small bowl, whisk together the olive oil, soy sauce, honey, and grated ginger.
3. Thread the shrimp and pineapple chunks onto skewers, alternating between the two.
4. Brush the skewers with the marinade.
5. Grill the skewers for 2-3 minutes per side, until the shrimp are pink and fully cooked.
6. Serve immediately.

Nutrition Info per Serving:
- Calories: 220
- Protein: 20g
- Carbohydrates: 15g
- Fat: 9g
- Fiber: 1g

Servings:
- Serves 4

Cooking Time:
- Total: 15 minutes

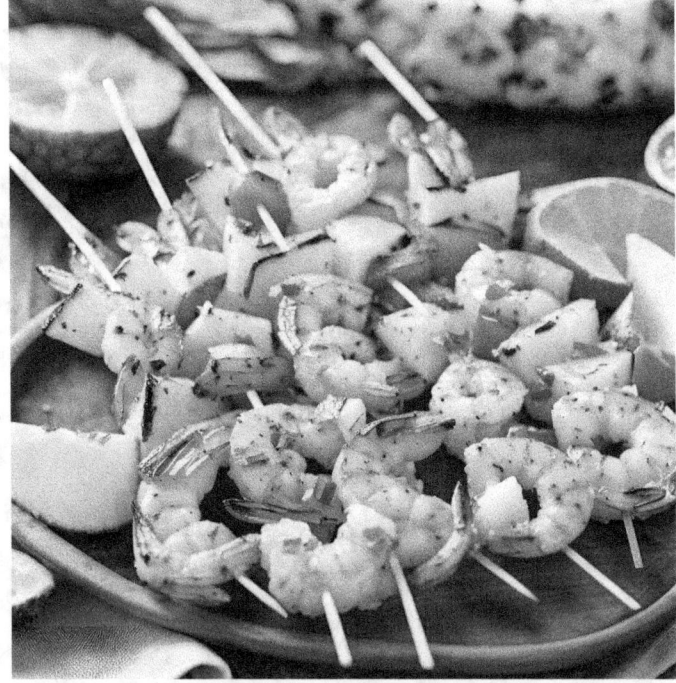

21. Squid Ink Pasta with Seafood

Ingredients:
- 8 oz squid ink pasta
- 2 tablespoons olive oil
- 1 small onion, finely chopped
- 2 cloves garlic, minced
- 1/2 pound shrimp, peeled and deveined
- 1/2 pound mussels, cleaned
- 1/2 pound squid rings
- 1/2 cup dry white wine (optional)
- 1 cup cherry tomatoes, halved
- 1/4 cup chopped fresh parsley
- 1 tablespoon lemon juice

Instructions:
1. Cook the squid ink pasta according to package instructions. Drain and set aside.
2. Heat the olive oil in a large skillet over medium heat.
3. Add the chopped onion and cook until softened, about 5 minutes.
4. Stir in the minced garlic and cook for another 1-2 minutes.
5. Add the shrimp, mussels, and squid rings to the skillet. Cook for 3-4 minutes until the shrimp are pink and the mussels have opened.
6. Pour in the white wine, if using, and cook for another 2 minutes until reduced.
7. Stir in the cherry tomatoes and cook for another 2 minutes.
8. Add the cooked pasta to the skillet and toss to combine.
9. Stir in the chopped parsley and lemon juice.
10. Serve immediately.

Nutrition Info per Serving:
- Calories: 400
- Protein: 30g
- Carbohydrates: 40g
- Fat: 12g
- Fiber: 4g

Servings:
- Serves 4

Cooking Time:
- **Total: 25 minutes**

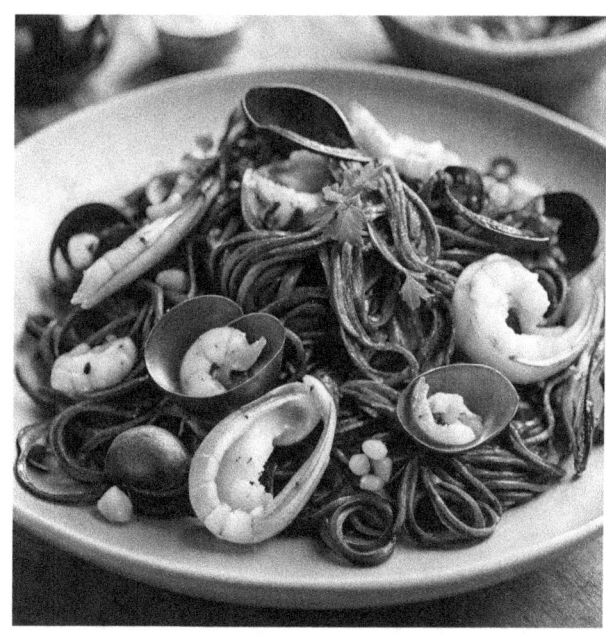

22. Lemon Pepper Haddock

Ingredients:
- 4 haddock fillets (about 6 oz each)
- 2 tablespoons olive oil
- 1 tablespoon lemon juice
- 1 teaspoon lemon zest
- 1 teaspoon garlic powder
- 1 teaspoon dried basil

Instructions:
1. Preheat the oven to 375°F (190°C).
2. Place the haddock fillets on a baking sheet lined with parchment paper.
3. In a small bowl, mix the olive oil, lemon juice, lemon zest, garlic powder, and dried basil.
4. Brush the mixture over the haddock fillets.
5. Bake for 15-20 minutes, or until the fish is fully cooked and flakes easily with a fork.
6. Serve immediately.

Nutrition Info per Serving:
- Calories: 250
- Protein: 28g
- Carbohydrates: 2g
- Fat: 14g
- Fiber: 0g

Servings:
- Serves 4

Cooking Time:
- **Total: 20 minutes**

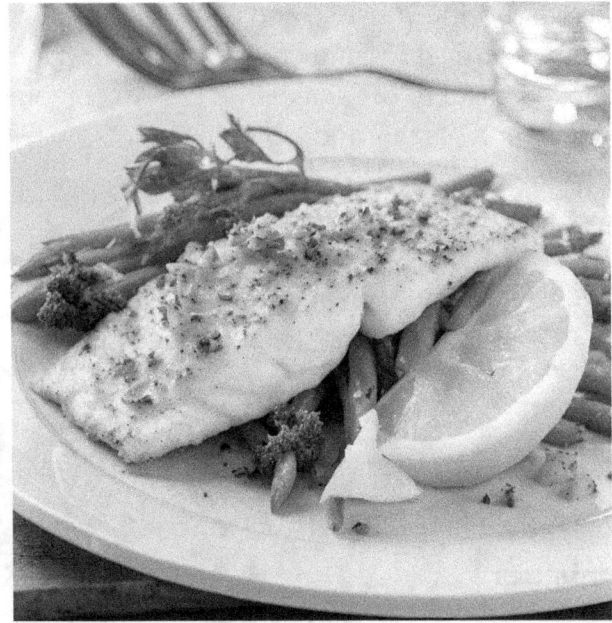

23. Bouillabaisse

Ingredients:
- 2 tablespoons olive oil
- 1 onion, finely chopped
- 2 leeks, white part only, thinly sliced
- 2 cloves garlic, minced
- 1 fennel bulb, thinly sliced
- 1 cup diced tomatoes
- 1/2 cup dry white wine (optional)
- 4 cups fish stock
- 1 teaspoon saffron threads
- 1/2 teaspoon dried thyme
- 1/2 teaspoon dried oregano
- 1 bay leaf
- 1 pound white fish fillets (such as cod or halibut), cut into chunks
- 1/2 pound mussels, cleaned
- 1/2 pound shrimp, peeled and deveined
- 1/2 pound squid rings
- 1/4 cup chopped fresh parsley
- 1 tablespoon lemon juice

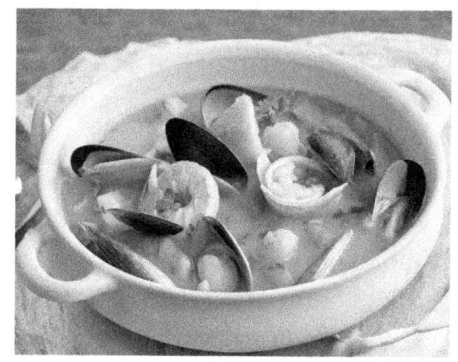

Instructions:
1. Heat the olive oil in a large pot over medium heat.
2. Add the chopped onion, sliced leeks, and fennel, and cook until softened, about 5 minutes.
3. Stir in the minced garlic and cook for another 1-2 minutes.
4. Add the diced tomatoes and cook for another 3-4 minutes.
5. Pour in the white wine, if using, and cook for 2-3 minutes until reduced.
6. Add the fish stock, saffron, dried thyme, dried oregano, and bay leaf. Bring to a boil, then reduce the heat and simmer for 20 minutes.
7. Add the white fish chunks, mussels, shrimp, and squid rings to the pot. Cook for 5-7 minutes, until the seafood is cooked through and the mussels have opened.
8. Stir in the chopped parsley and lemon juice.
9. Serve immediately.

Nutrition Info per Serving:
- Calories: 300   Protein: 32g   Carbohydrates: 12g   Fat: 12g   Fiber: 3g

Servings:
- Serves 6

Cooking Time:
- Total: 45 minutes

24. Seared Scallops with Mango Salsa

Ingredients:
- 1 pound sea scallops
- 2 tablespoons olive oil
- 1 mango, peeled and diced
- 1/2 red bell pepper, diced
- 1/4 red onion, finely chopped
- 1 tablespoon lime juice
- 1 tablespoon chopped fresh cilantro
- 1 teaspoon grated fresh ginger

Instructions:
1. Pat the scallops dry with paper towels.
2. Heat the olive oil in a large skillet over medium-high heat.
3. Add the scallops to the skillet and cook for 2-3 minutes per side, until golden brown and cooked through. Remove from the skillet and set aside.
4. In a medium bowl, combine the diced mango, red bell pepper, red onion, lime juice, chopped cilantro, and grated ginger. Mix well.
5. Serve the seared scallops topped with the mango salsa.

Nutrition Info per Serving:
- Calories: 240
- Protein: 24g
- Carbohydrates: 16g
- Fat: 10g
- Fiber: 2g

Servings:
- Serves 4

Cooking Time:
- Total: 15 minutes

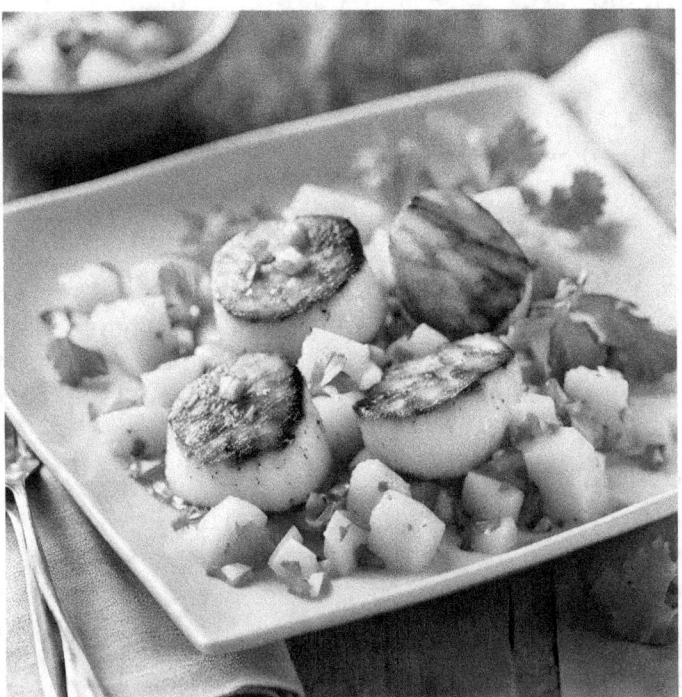

25. Anchovy and Broccoli Pasta

Ingredients:
- 8 oz whole wheat pasta
- 2 tablespoons olive oil
- 4 anchovy fillets, minced
- 3 cloves garlic, minced
- 1/4 teaspoon red pepper flakes (optional)
- 1 large head of broccoli, cut into small florets
- 1/4 cup grated Parmesan cheese
- 1 tablespoon lemon juice
- 1/4 cup chopped fresh parsley

Instructions:
1. Cook the pasta according to package instructions. Drain and set aside.
2. In a large skillet, heat the olive oil over medium heat.
3. Add the minced anchovy fillets, minced garlic, and red pepper flakes, if using. Cook for 1-2 minutes until fragrant.
4. Add the broccoli florets to the skillet and cook for 5-7 minutes until tender.
5. Add the cooked pasta to the skillet and toss to combine.
6. Stir in the grated Parmesan cheese and lemon juice.
7. Garnish with chopped fresh parsley before serving.

Nutrition Info per Serving:
- Calories: 350
- Protein: 15g
- Carbohydrates: 50g
- Fat: 12g
- Fiber: 8g

Servings:
- Serves 4

Cooking Time:
- **Total: 20 minutes**

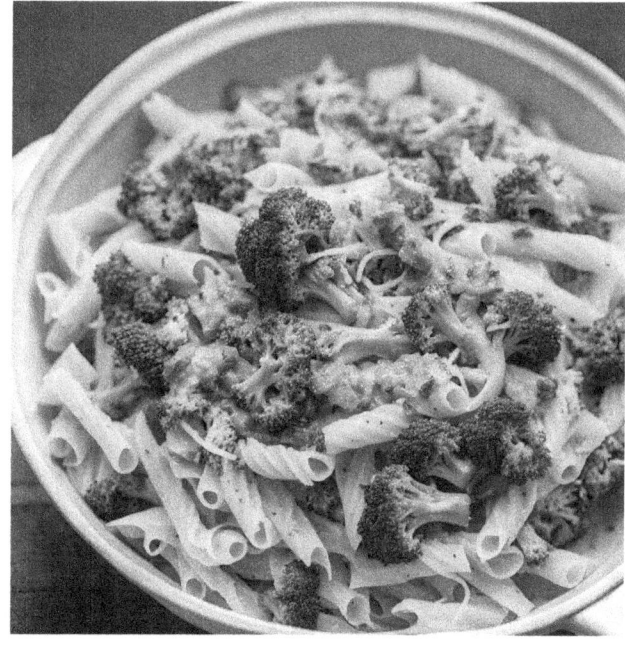

Vegetables

1. Roasted Cauliflower with Turmeric and Cumin

Ingredients:
- 1 large head of cauliflower, cut into florets
- 3 tablespoons olive oil
- 1 teaspoon ground turmeric
- 1 teaspoon ground cumin
- 1 teaspoon garlic powder
- 1 tablespoon lemon juice
- 2 tablespoons chopped fresh cilantro (optional)

Instructions:
1. Preheat the oven to 400°F (200°C).
2. In a large bowl, toss the cauliflower florets with olive oil, turmeric, cumin, garlic powder, and lemon juice until well coated.
3. Spread the cauliflower florets in a single layer on a baking sheet.
4. Roast in the preheated oven for 25-30 minutes, stirring halfway through, until the cauliflower is golden brown and tender.
5. Garnish with chopped fresh cilantro before serving, if desired.

Nutrition Info per Serving:
- Calories: 150
- Protein: 3g
- Carbohydrates: 12g
- Fat: 10g
- Fiber: 5g

Servings:
- Serves 4

Cooking Time:
- Total: 35 minutes

2. Kale and Quinoa Salad with Lemon Vinaigrette

Ingredients:
- 1 cup quinoa, rinsed
- 2 cups water
- 4 cups chopped kale
- 1/2 cup shredded carrots
- 1/4 cup chopped red onion
- 1/4 cup chopped walnuts
- 1/4 cup dried cranberries
- 1/4 cup olive oil
- 2 tablespoons lemon juice
- 1 teaspoon Dijon mustard
- 1 teaspoon honey

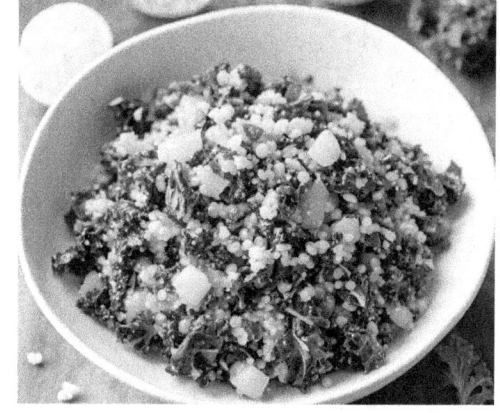

Instructions:
1. In a medium saucepan, bring the quinoa and water to a boil. Reduce the heat to low, cover, and simmer for 15 minutes or until the quinoa is tender and the water is absorbed. Fluff with a fork and let cool.
2. In a large bowl, combine the chopped kale, shredded carrots, chopped red onion, chopped walnuts, and dried cranberries.
3. Add the cooled quinoa to the bowl.
4. In a small bowl, whisk together the olive oil, lemon juice, Dijon mustard, and honey to make the vinaigrette.
5. Pour the vinaigrette over the salad and toss to combine.
6. Serve immediately or refrigerate until ready to eat.

Nutrition Info per Serving:
- Calories: 280
- Protein: 6g
- Carbohydrates: 30g
- Fat: 16g
- Fiber: 5g

Servings:
- Serves 4

Cooking Time:
- **Total: 20 minutes (plus cooling time for quinoa)**

3. Stuffed Bell Peppers with Brown Rice and Vegetables

Ingredients:
- 4 large bell peppers, tops cut off and seeds removed
- 1 cup cooked brown rice
- 1 cup black beans, drained and rinsed
- 1 cup corn kernels (fresh or frozen)
- 1/2 cup diced tomatoes
- 1/2 cup diced onion
- 1/2 cup shredded cheddar cheese
- 2 tablespoons olive oil
- 1 teaspoon ground cumin
- 1 teaspoon garlic powder
- 1/4 cup chopped fresh cilantro (optional)

Instructions:
1. Preheat the oven to 375°F (190°C).
2. In a large skillet, heat the olive oil over medium heat.
3. Add the diced onion and cook until softened, about 5 minutes.
4. Stir in the ground cumin and garlic powder, cooking for another minute.
5. Add the cooked brown rice, black beans, corn kernels, and diced tomatoes to the skillet. Cook for 5 minutes, stirring occasionally, until heated through.
6. Remove from heat and stir in the shredded cheddar cheese.
7. Stuff the bell peppers with the rice and vegetable mixture, pressing down gently to fill them completely.
8. Place the stuffed peppers in a baking dish and cover with foil.
9. Bake in the preheated oven for 25-30 minutes, until the peppers are tender.
10. Garnish with chopped fresh cilantro before serving, if desired.

Nutrition Info per Serving:
- Calories: 350
- Protein: 10g
- Carbohydrates: 45g
- Fat: 15g
- Fiber: 8g

Servings:
- Serves 4

Cooking Time:
- Total: 40 minutes

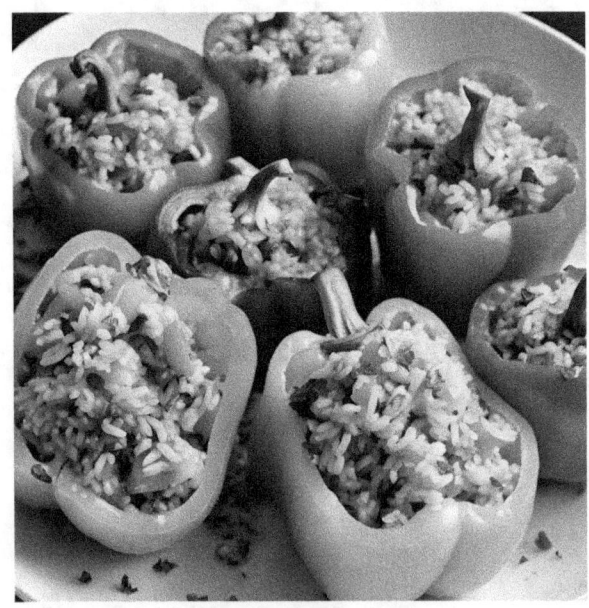

4. Spicy Roasted Sweet Potatoes

Ingredients:
- 2 large sweet potatoes, peeled and cut into cubes
- 3 tablespoons olive oil
- 1 teaspoon ground cumin
- 1 teaspoon smoked paprika
- 1/2 teaspoon cayenne pepper (adjust to taste)
- 1 teaspoon garlic powder
- 1 tablespoon lime juice
- 2 tablespoons chopped fresh parsley (optional)

Instructions:
1. Preheat the oven to 425°F (220°C).
2. In a large bowl, toss the sweet potato cubes with olive oil, cumin, smoked paprika, cayenne pepper, garlic powder, and lime juice until well coated.
3. Spread the sweet potato cubes in a single layer on a baking sheet.
4. Roast in the preheated oven for 25-30 minutes, stirring halfway through, until the sweet potatoes are golden brown and tender.
5. Garnish with chopped fresh parsley before serving, if desired.

Nutrition Info per Serving:
- Calories: 200
- Protein: 2g
- Carbohydrates: 30g
- Fat: 10g
- Fiber: 5g

Servings:
- Serves 4

Cooking Time:
- **Total: 35 minutes**

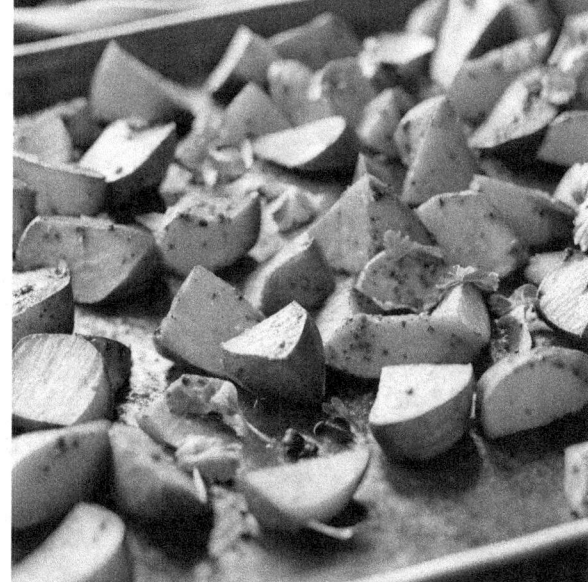

5. Zucchini Noodles with Pesto and Cherry Tomatoes

Ingredients:
- 4 medium zucchinis, spiralized into noodles
- 1 cup cherry tomatoes, halved
- 1/4 cup basil pesto
- 2 tablespoons olive oil
- 1/4 cup grated Parmesan cheese
- 1/4 cup chopped fresh basil

Instructions:
1. Heat the olive oil in a large skillet over medium heat.
2. Add the zucchini noodles and cook for 3-4 minutes, until just tender.
3. Stir in the basil pesto and cook for another 2 minutes.
4. Add the cherry tomatoes and cook for 1-2 minutes, until warmed through.
5. Remove from heat and toss with grated Parmesan cheese.
6. Garnish with chopped fresh basil before serving.

Nutrition Info per Serving:
- Calories: 200
- Protein: 6g
- Carbohydrates: 10g
- Fat: 16g
- Fiber: 3g

Servings:
- Serves 4

Cooking Time:
- **Total: 10 minutes**

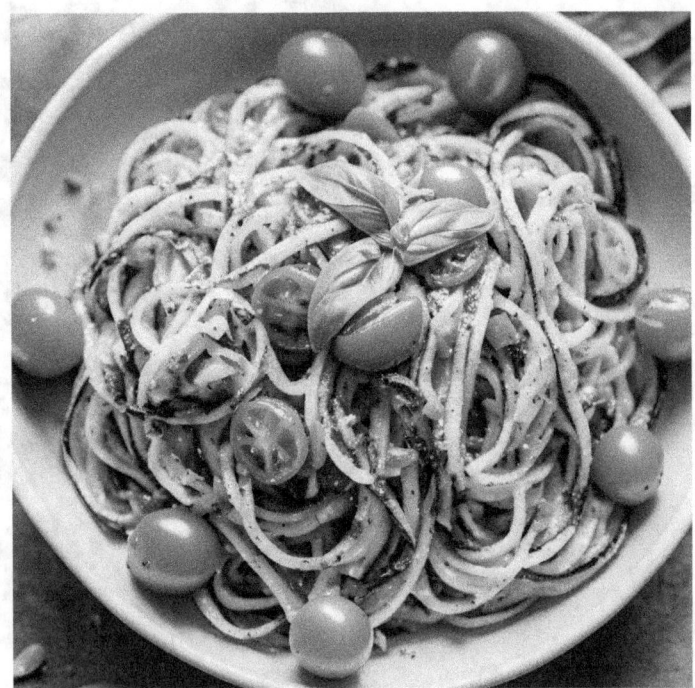

6. Grilled Eggplant with Tahini Sauce

Ingredients:
- 2 large eggplants, sliced into rounds
- 3 tablespoons olive oil
- 1/4 cup tahini
- 2 tablespoons lemon juice
- 1 clove garlic, minced
- 2 tablespoons water
- 1/4 cup chopped fresh parsley

Instructions:
1. Preheat the grill to medium-high heat.
2. Brush the eggplant slices with olive oil on both sides.
3. Grill the eggplant slices for 3-4 minutes per side, until tender and grill marks appear.
4. While the eggplant is grilling, prepare the tahini sauce. In a small bowl, whisk together the tahini, lemon juice, minced garlic, and water until smooth.
5. Arrange the grilled eggplant slices on a serving platter and drizzle with the tahini sauce.
6. Garnish with chopped fresh parsley before serving.

Nutrition Info per Serving:
- Calories: 220
- Protein: 4g
- Carbohydrates: 12g
- Fat: 18g
- Fiber: 6g

Servings:
- Serves 4

Cooking Time:
- **Total: 15 minutes**

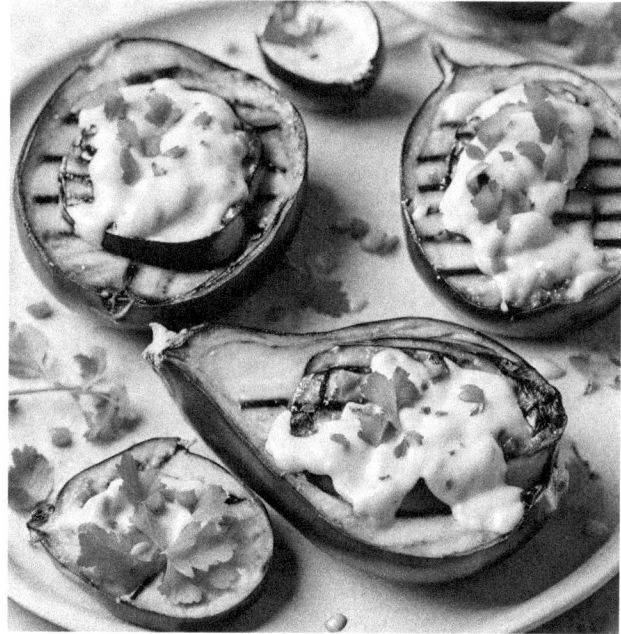

7. Beetroot and Feta Salad

Ingredients:
- 4 medium beetroots, roasted and diced
- 1/4 cup crumbled feta cheese
- 1/4 cup chopped walnuts
- 2 cups mixed salad greens
- 2 tablespoons olive oil
- 1 tablespoon balsamic vinegar
- 1 teaspoon honey

Instructions:
1. Preheat the oven to 400°F (200°C).
2. Wrap the beetroots in aluminum foil and roast in the oven for 45-60 minutes, until tender. Let cool, then peel and dice.
3. In a large bowl, combine the diced beetroots, crumbled feta cheese, chopped walnuts, and mixed salad greens.
4. In a small bowl, whisk together the olive oil, balsamic vinegar, and honey to make the dressing.
5. Pour the dressing over the salad and toss to combine.
6. Serve immediately.

Nutrition Info per Serving:
- Calories: 250
- Protein: 6g
- Carbohydrates: 20g
- Fat: 18g
- Fiber: 5g

Servings:
- Serves 4

Cooking Time:
- **Total: 1 hour**

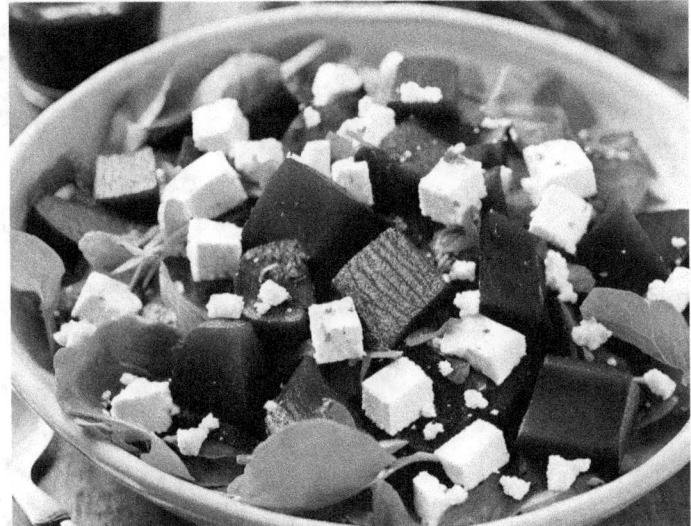

8. Broccoli and Almond Stir-Fry

Ingredients:
- 4 cups broccoli florets
- 1 red bell pepper, sliced
- 2 tablespoons olive oil
- 2 cloves garlic, minced
- 1/4 cup sliced almonds
- 2 tablespoons low-sodium soy sauce
- 1 tablespoon sesame oil
- 1 teaspoon grated fresh ginger

Instructions:
1. Heat the olive oil in a large skillet or wok over medium-high heat.
2. Add the minced garlic and grated ginger, cooking for 1 minute until fragrant.
3. Add the broccoli florets and red bell pepper, stir-frying for 5-7 minutes until tender-crisp.
4. Stir in the low-sodium soy sauce and sesame oil, cooking for another 2 minutes.
5. Remove from heat and toss with sliced almonds.
6. Serve immediately.

Nutrition Info per Serving:
- Calories: 180
- Protein: 5g
- Carbohydrates: 12g
- Fat: 14g
- Fiber: 5g

Servings:
- Serves 4

Cooking Time:
- **Total: 15 minutes**

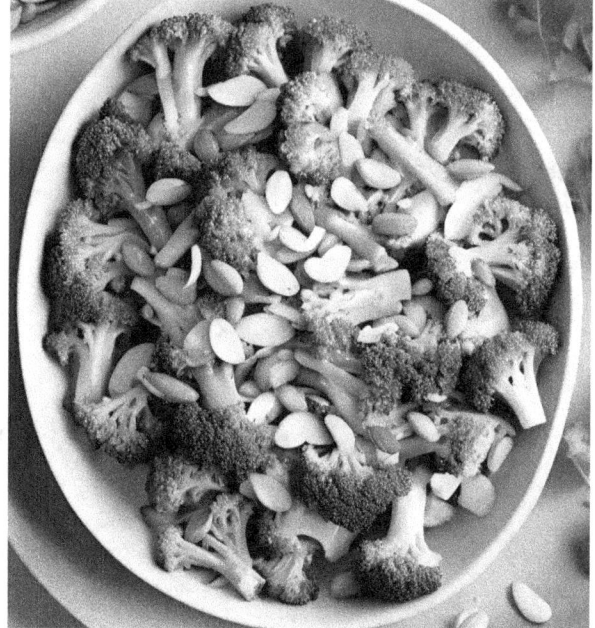

9. Spinach and Mushroom Quiche

Ingredients:
- 1 pre-made pie crust
- 2 tablespoons olive oil
- 1 small onion, diced
- 2 cloves garlic, minced
- 2 cups fresh spinach, chopped
- 1 cup sliced mushrooms
- 4 large eggs
- 1 cup milk (or dairy-free alternative)
- 1/2 cup shredded Swiss cheese
- 1/4 teaspoon ground nutmeg

Instructions:
1. Preheat the oven to 375°F (190°C).
2. Place the pie crust in a pie dish and set aside.
3. Heat the olive oil in a skillet over medium heat.
4. Add the diced onion and minced garlic, cooking until softened, about 5 minutes.
5. Stir in the chopped spinach and sliced mushrooms, cooking until the spinach is wilted and the mushrooms are tender, about 3-4 minutes.
6. In a medium bowl, whisk together the eggs, milk, shredded Swiss cheese, and ground nutmeg.
7. Spread the spinach and mushroom mixture evenly in the pie crust.
8. Pour the egg mixture over the vegetables.
9. Bake for 35-40 minutes, or until the quiche is set and golden brown.
10. Allow to cool slightly before slicing and serving.

Nutrition Info per Serving:
- Calories: 280
- Protein: 10g
- Carbohydrates: 22g
- Fat: 18g
- Fiber: 2g

Servings:
- Serves 6

Cooking Time:
- **Total: 50 minutes**

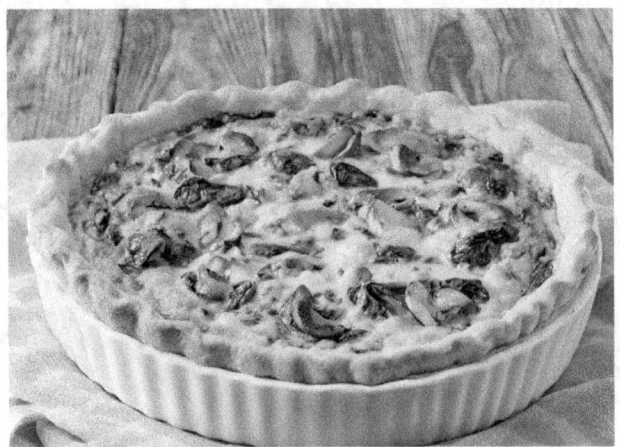

10. Cabbage Slaw with Apple Cider Vinegar Dressing

Ingredients:
- 4 cups shredded green cabbage
- 1 cup shredded red cabbage
- 1 cup shredded carrots
- 1/2 cup chopped fresh parsley
- 1/4 cup apple cider vinegar
- 2 tablespoons olive oil
- 1 tablespoon honey
- 1 teaspoon Dijon mustard

Instructions:
1. In a large bowl, combine the shredded green cabbage, red cabbage, carrots, and chopped parsley.
2. In a small bowl, whisk together the apple cider vinegar, olive oil, honey, and Dijon mustard to make the dressing.
3. Pour the dressing over the cabbage mixture and toss to combine.
4. Refrigerate for at least 30 minutes before serving to allow the flavors to meld.

Nutrition Info per Serving:
- Calories: 90
- Protein: 1g
- Carbohydrates: 10g
- Fat: 5g
- Fiber: 3g

Servings:
- Serves 6

Cooking Time:
- **Total: 10 minutes (plus 30 minutes refrigeration)**

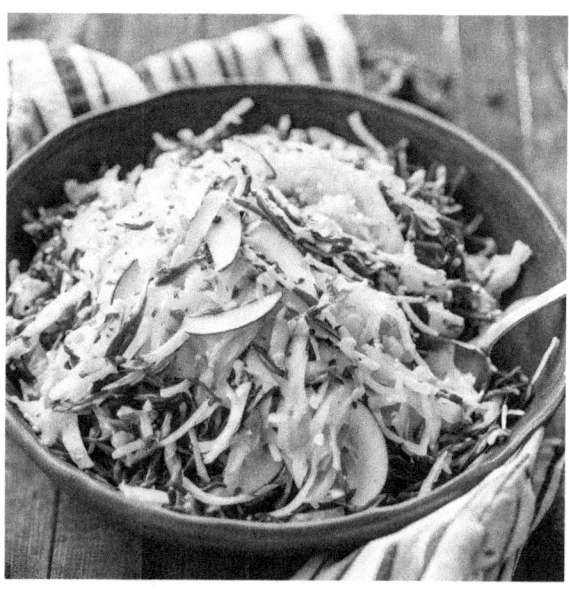

11. Asparagus and Feta Omelette

Ingredients:
- 6 large eggs
- 1/4 cup milk (or dairy-free alternative)
- 1 tablespoon olive oil
- 1 cup asparagus, cut into 1-inch pieces
- 1/4 cup crumbled feta cheese
- 1/2 teaspoon dried oregano

Instructions:
1. In a medium bowl, whisk together the eggs and milk until well combined.
2. Heat the olive oil in a non-stick skillet over medium heat.
3. Add the asparagus and cook for 3-4 minutes until tender.
4. Pour the egg mixture into the skillet, covering the asparagus.
5. Cook for 2-3 minutes until the edges start to set, then sprinkle the crumbled feta cheese and dried oregano over the top.
6. Fold the omelette in half and cook for another 1-2 minutes until fully set.
7. Serve immediately.

Nutrition Info per Serving:
- Calories: 200
- Protein: 12g
- Carbohydrates: 4g
- Fat: 15g
- Fiber: 1g

Servings:
- Serves 2

Cooking Time:
- Total: 10 minutes

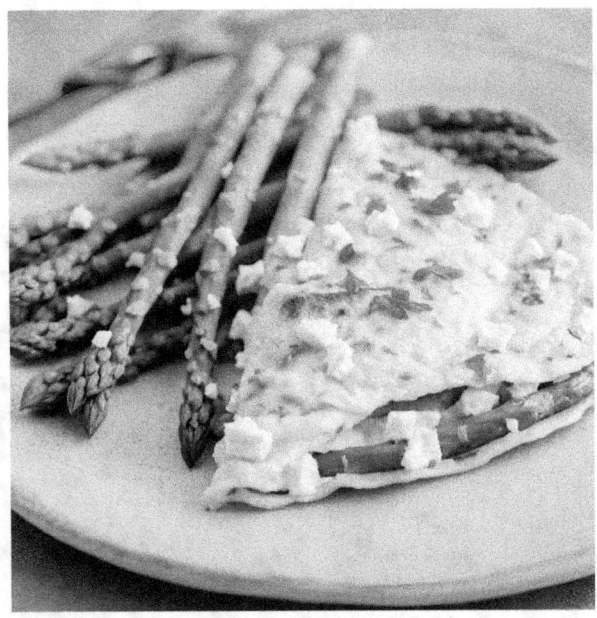

12. Butternut Squash Risotto

Ingredients:
- 1 tablespoon olive oil
- 1 small onion, finely chopped
- 2 cloves garlic, minced
- 1 cup Arborio rice
- 1 cup diced butternut squash
- 4 cups low-sodium vegetable broth, warmed
- 1/2 cup grated Parmesan cheese
- 1 tablespoon chopped fresh sage
- 1 tablespoon butter (optional)

Instructions:
1. Heat the olive oil in a large saucepan over medium heat.
2. Add the chopped onion and cook until softened, about 5 minutes.
3. Stir in the minced garlic and Arborio rice, cooking for 1-2 minutes until the rice is lightly toasted.
4. Add the diced butternut squash and cook for another 2 minutes.
5. Gradually add the warmed vegetable broth, one ladle at a time, stirring frequently and allowing the liquid to be absorbed before adding more. Continue this process until the rice is creamy and tender, about 18-20 minutes.
6. Stir in the grated Parmesan cheese, chopped fresh sage, and butter (if using).
7. Serve immediately.

Nutrition Info per Serving:
- Calories: 320
- Protein: 8g
- Carbohydrates: 50g
- Fat: 10g
- Fiber: 3g

Servings:
- Serves 4

Cooking Time:
- **Total: 30 minutes**

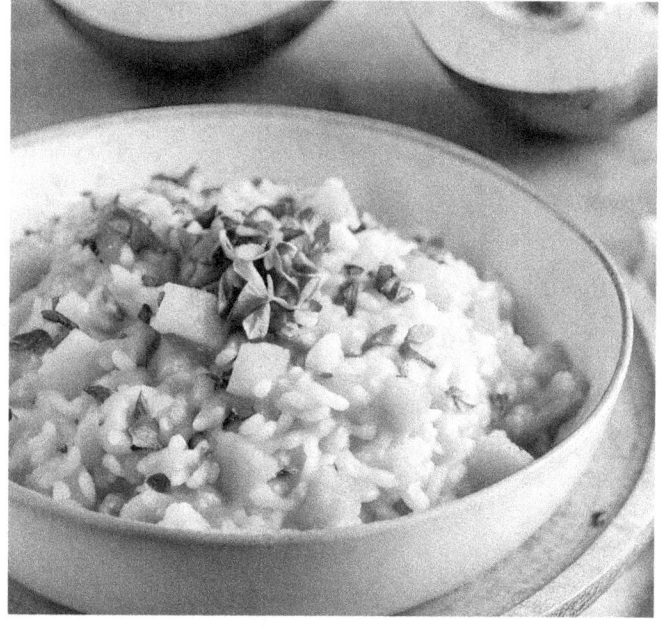

13. Vegetable Paella with Saffron

Ingredients:
- 2 tablespoons olive oil
- 1 onion, finely chopped
- 2 cloves garlic, minced
- 1 red bell pepper, sliced
- 1 yellow bell pepper, sliced
- 1 cup Arborio rice
- 1/2 teaspoon saffron threads
- 1 can (14.5 oz) diced tomatoes
- 4 cups low-sodium vegetable broth
- 1 cup green beans, trimmed and cut into 1-inch pieces
- 1 cup frozen peas
- 1/4 cup chopped fresh parsley
- 1 tablespoon lemon juice

Instructions:
1. Heat the olive oil in a large skillet or paella pan over medium heat.
2. Add the chopped onion and cook until softened, about 5 minutes.
3. Stir in the minced garlic, red bell pepper, and yellow bell pepper, cooking for another 5 minutes until tender.
4. Add the Arborio rice and saffron threads, stirring to coat the rice with the oil.
5. Pour in the diced tomatoes and vegetable broth, stirring to combine.
6. Bring to a simmer and cook for 15 minutes, stirring occasionally.
7. Add the green beans and cook for another 10 minutes.
8. Stir in the frozen peas and cook for an additional 2 minutes.
9. Remove from heat and stir in the chopped fresh parsley and lemon juice.
10. Serve immediately.

Nutrition Info per Serving:
- Calories: 280
- Protein: 7g
- Carbohydrates: 45g
- Fat: 8g
- Fiber: 6g

Servings:
- Serves 4

Cooking Time:
- **Total: 35 minutes**

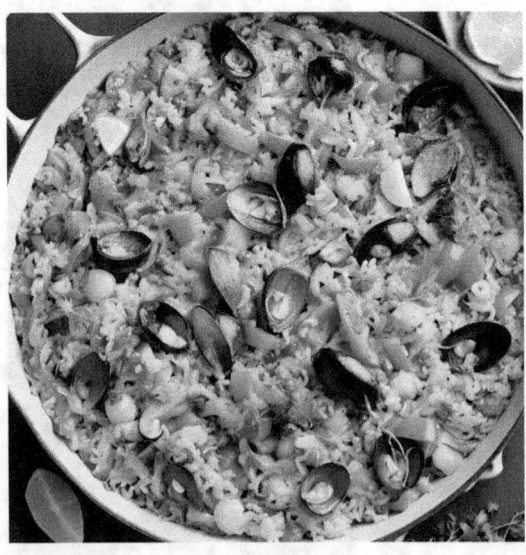

14. Stir-Fried Bok Choy with Garlic and Soy Sauce

Ingredients:
- 1 tablespoon olive oil
- 2 cloves garlic, minced
- 1 pound bok choy, chopped
- 2 tablespoons low-sodium soy sauce
- 1 teaspoon sesame oil
- 1 teaspoon grated fresh ginger

Instructions:
1. Heat the olive oil in a large skillet or wok over medium-high heat.
2. Add the minced garlic and grated fresh ginger, cooking for 1 minute until fragrant.
3. Add the chopped bok choy and stir-fry for 5-7 minutes until tender.
4. Stir in the low-sodium soy sauce and sesame oil, cooking for another 2 minutes.
5. Serve immediately.

Nutrition Info per Serving:
- Calories: 100
- Protein: 4g
- Carbohydrates: 10g
- Fat: 6g
- Fiber: 3g

Servings:
- Serves 4

Cooking Time:
- **Total: 15 minutes**

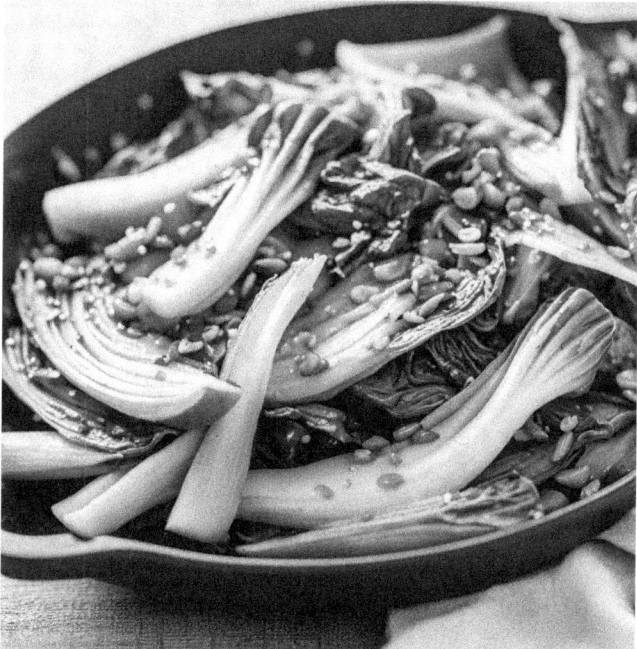

15. Cucumber and Dill Salad with Yogurt Dressing

Ingredients:
- 2 large cucumbers, thinly sliced
- 1/4 cup red onion, thinly sliced
- 1/4 cup fresh dill, chopped
- 1 cup plain Greek yogurt
- 2 tablespoons lemon juice
- 1 teaspoon garlic powder

Instructions:
1. In a large bowl, combine the sliced cucumbers, red onion, and chopped dill.
2. In a separate small bowl, whisk together the Greek yogurt, lemon juice, and garlic powder to make the dressing.
3. Pour the yogurt dressing over the cucumber mixture and toss to coat evenly.
4. Refrigerate for at least 30 minutes before serving to allow the flavors to meld.

Nutrition Info per Serving:
- Calories: 80
- Protein: 5g
- Carbohydrates: 10g
- Fat: 3g
- Fiber: 2g

Servings:
- Serves 4

Cooking Time:
- **Total: 10 minutes (plus 30 minutes refrigeration)**

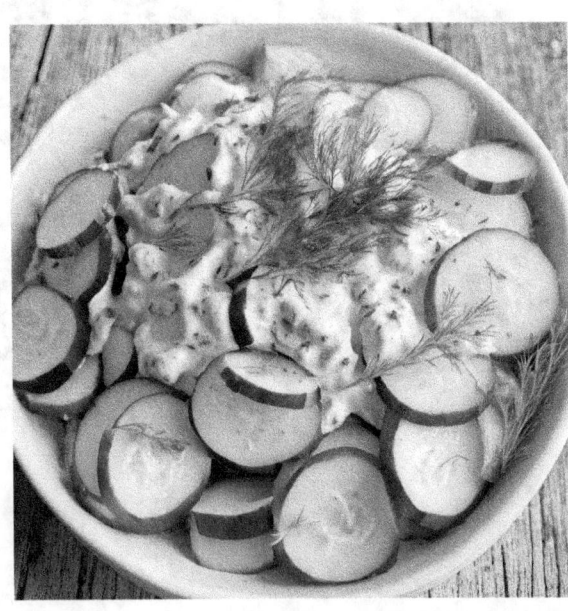

16. Tomato Gazpacho

Ingredients:
- 4 large tomatoes, chopped
- 1 cucumber, peeled and chopped
- 1 red bell pepper, chopped
- 1 small red onion, chopped
- 2 cloves garlic, minced
- 2 cups tomato juice
- 2 tablespoons olive oil
- 2 tablespoons red wine vinegar
- 1 teaspoon cumin
- 1/4 cup chopped fresh basil

Instructions:
1. In a blender or food processor, combine the chopped tomatoes, cucumber, red bell pepper, red onion, and garlic. Blend until smooth.
2. Transfer the mixture to a large bowl and stir in the tomato juice, olive oil, red wine vinegar, and cumin.
3. Refrigerate for at least 1 hour before serving to allow the flavors to meld.
4. Garnish with chopped fresh basil before serving.

Nutrition Info per Serving:
- Calories: 120
- Protein: 2g
- Carbohydrates: 15g
- Fat: 7g
- Fiber: 3g

Servings:
- Serves 4

Cooking Time:
- Total: 15 minutes (plus 1 hour refrigeration)

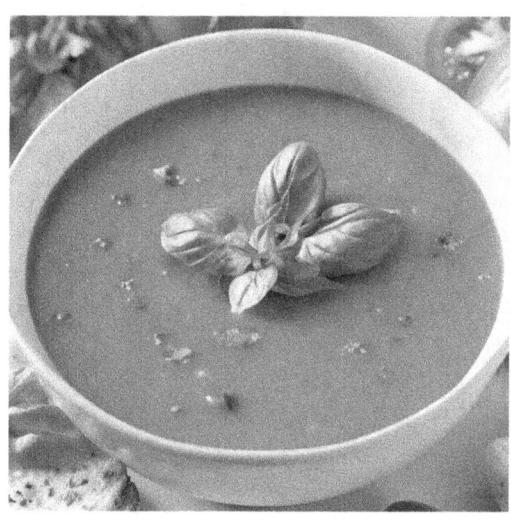

17. Mushroom and Barley Soup

Ingredients:
- 2 tablespoons olive oil
- 1 onion, finely chopped
- 2 cloves garlic, minced
- 1 pound mushrooms, sliced
- 1 cup pearl barley
- 6 cups vegetable broth
- 2 carrots, sliced
- 2 celery stalks, sliced
- 1 teaspoon dried thyme
- 1 bay leaf
- 1/4 cup chopped fresh parsley

Instructions:
1. Heat the olive oil in a large pot over medium heat.
2. Add the chopped onion and cook until softened, about 5 minutes.
3. Stir in the minced garlic and sliced mushrooms, cooking for another 5 minutes until the mushrooms are tender.
4. Add the pearl barley, vegetable broth, sliced carrots, sliced celery, dried thyme, and bay leaf. Bring to a boil.
5. Reduce the heat and simmer for 30-40 minutes, until the barley is tender.
6. Remove the bay leaf and stir in the chopped fresh parsley before serving.

Nutrition Info per Serving:
- Calories: 200
- Protein: 6g
- Carbohydrates: 35g
- Fat: 6g
- Fiber: 8g

Servings:
- Serves 6

Cooking Time:
- **Total: 50 minutes**

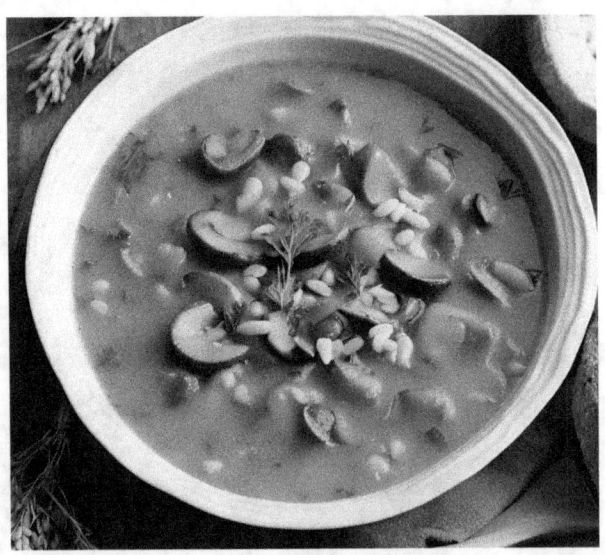

18. Curried Lentils with Spinach and Carrots

Ingredients:
- 2 tablespoons olive oil
- 1 onion, finely chopped
- 2 cloves garlic, minced
- 1 tablespoon grated fresh ginger
- 1 tablespoon curry powder
- 1 cup dried lentils, rinsed
- 4 cups vegetable broth
- 2 carrots, sliced
- 4 cups fresh spinach
- 1/4 cup coconut milk
- 1 tablespoon lemon juice

Instructions:
1. Heat the olive oil in a large pot over medium heat.
2. Add the chopped onion and cook until softened, about 5 minutes.
3. Stir in the minced garlic, grated ginger, and curry powder, cooking for another 1-2 minutes until fragrant.
4. Add the rinsed lentils, vegetable broth, and sliced carrots. Bring to a boil.
5. Reduce the heat and simmer for 20-25 minutes, until the lentils are tender.
6. Stir in the fresh spinach and cook until wilted, about 2 minutes.
7. Remove from heat and stir in the coconut milk and lemon juice.
8. Serve immediately.

Nutrition Info per Serving:
- Calories: 250
- Protein: 12g
- Carbohydrates: 35g
- Fat: 8g
- Fiber: 12g

Servings:
- Serves 4

Cooking Time:
- **Total: 35 minutes**

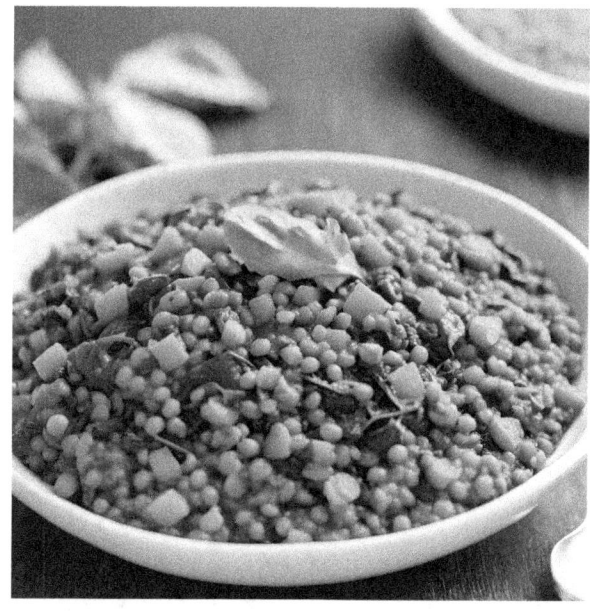

19. Sweet Potato and Chickpea Curry

Ingredients:
- 2 tablespoons olive oil
- 1 onion, finely chopped
- 2 cloves garlic, minced
- 1 tablespoon grated fresh ginger
- 1 tablespoon curry powder
- 1 teaspoon ground cumin
- 1 teaspoon turmeric
- 2 medium sweet potatoes, peeled and cubed
- 1 can (15 oz) chickpeas, drained and rinsed
- 1 can (14 oz) diced tomatoes
- 1 can (14 oz) coconut milk
- 2 cups vegetable broth
- 2 cups fresh spinach
- 1 tablespoon lemon juice

Instructions:
1. Heat the olive oil in a large pot over medium heat.
2. Add the chopped onion and cook until softened, about 5 minutes.
3. Stir in the minced garlic, grated ginger, curry powder, ground cumin, and turmeric, cooking for another 1-2 minutes until fragrant.
4. Add the cubed sweet potatoes, chickpeas, diced tomatoes, coconut milk, and vegetable broth. Bring to a boil.
5. Reduce the heat and simmer for 20-25 minutes, until the sweet potatoes are tender.
6. Stir in the fresh spinach and cook until wilted, about 2 minutes.
7. Remove from heat and stir in the lemon juice.
8. Serve immediately.

Nutrition Info per Serving:
- Calories: 350
- Protein: 8g
- Carbohydrates: 50g
- Fat: 14g
- Fiber: 10g

Servings:
- Serves 4

Cooking Time:
- **Total: 35 minutes**

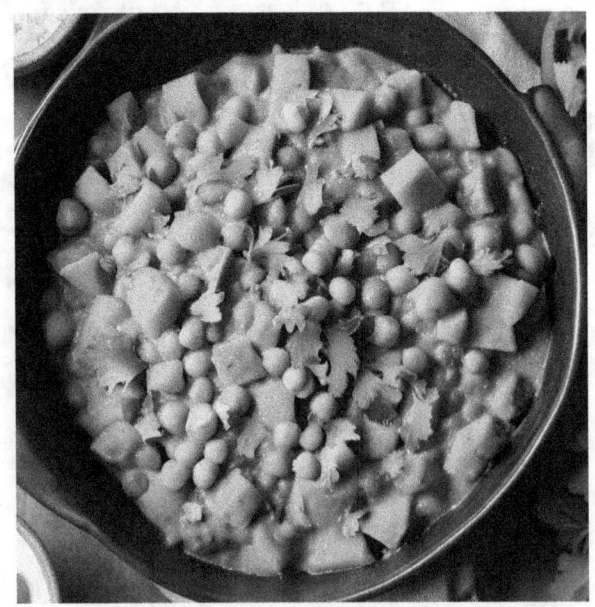

20. Roasted Parsnips and Carrots with Honey Glaze

Ingredients:
- 4 large parsnips, peeled and cut into sticks
- 4 large carrots, peeled and cut into sticks
- 3 tablespoons olive oil
- 2 tablespoons honey
- 1 teaspoon ground cumin
- 1 teaspoon dried thyme
- 1 tablespoon lemon juice

Instructions:
1. Preheat the oven to 400°F (200°C).
2. In a large bowl, toss the parsnips and carrots with olive oil, honey, ground cumin, and dried thyme until well coated.
3. Spread the vegetables in a single layer on a baking sheet.
4. Roast in the preheated oven for 25-30 minutes, stirring halfway through, until the vegetables are tender and golden brown.
5. Remove from the oven and drizzle with lemon juice before serving.

Nutrition Info per Serving:
- Calories: 180
- Protein: 2g
- Carbohydrates: 30g
- Fat: 7g
- Fiber: 6g

Servings:
- Serves 4

Cooking Time:
- **Total: 35 minutes**

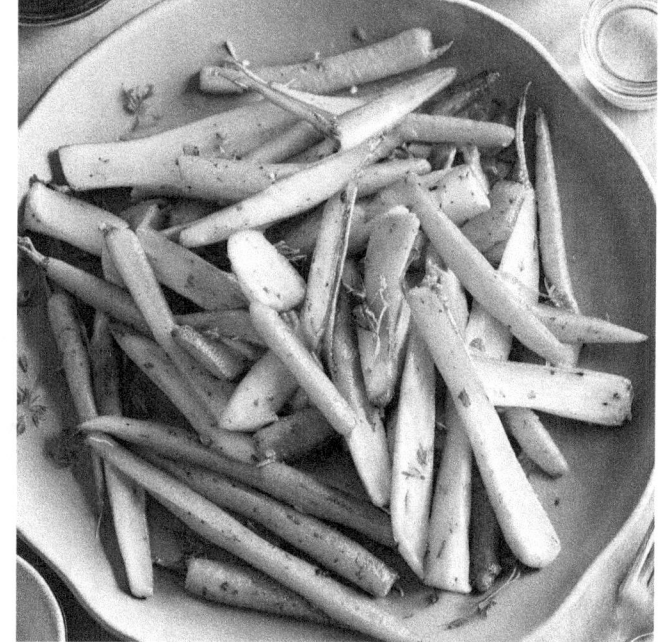

21. Creamy Avocado Spinach Pasta

Ingredients:
- 8 oz whole wheat pasta
- 2 tablespoons olive oil
- 2 cloves garlic, minced
- 4 cups fresh spinach
- 1 ripe avocado, peeled and pitted
- 1/4 cup plain Greek yogurt
- 1/4 cup grated Parmesan cheese
- 1 tablespoon lemon juice
- 1/4 cup chopped fresh basil

Instructions:
1. Cook the pasta according to package instructions. Drain and set aside.
2. In a large skillet, heat the olive oil over medium heat.
3. Add the minced garlic and cook for 1-2 minutes until fragrant.
4. Add the fresh spinach and cook until wilted, about 3-4 minutes.
5. In a blender or food processor, combine the avocado, Greek yogurt, grated Parmesan cheese, and lemon juice. Blend until smooth.
6. Add the cooked pasta and avocado sauce to the skillet with the spinach. Toss to combine and heat through.
7. Garnish with chopped fresh basil before serving.

Nutrition Info per Serving:
- Calories: 350
- Protein: 12g
- Carbohydrates: 45g
- Fat: 14g
- Fiber: 8g

Servings:
- Serves 4

Cooking Time:
- **Total: 20 minutes**

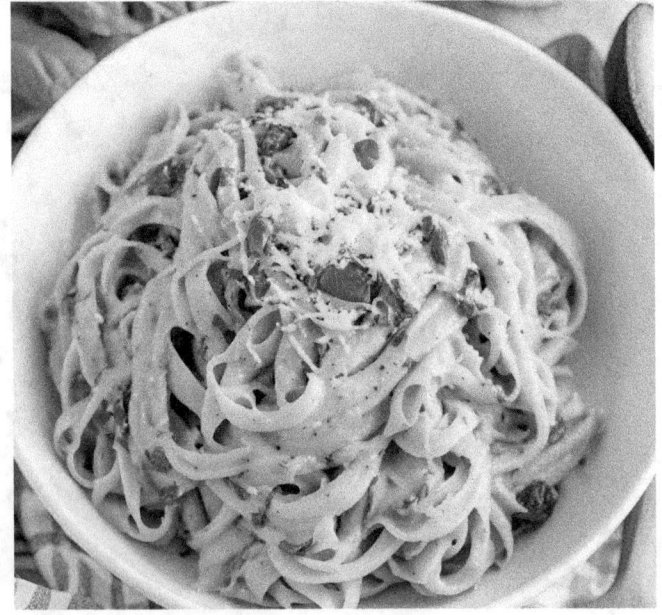

22. Vegan Cauliflower Tacos

Ingredients:
- 1 large head of cauliflower, cut into florets
- 3 tablespoons olive oil
- 1 tablespoon ground cumin
- 1 tablespoon smoked paprika
- 1 teaspoon garlic powder
- 8 small corn tortillas
- 1 cup shredded red cabbage
- 1/4 cup chopped fresh cilantro
- 1 avocado, sliced
- 1 lime, cut into wedges

Instructions:
1. Preheat the oven to 400°F (200°C).
2. In a large bowl, toss the cauliflower florets with olive oil, ground cumin, smoked paprika, and garlic powder until well coated.
3. Spread the cauliflower florets in a single layer on a baking sheet.
4. Roast in the preheated oven for 25-30 minutes, stirring halfway through, until the cauliflower is tender and golden brown.
5. Warm the corn tortillas in a skillet or microwave.
6. Assemble the tacos by placing roasted cauliflower in each tortilla and topping with shredded red cabbage, chopped fresh cilantro, and sliced avocado.
7. Serve with lime wedges on the side.

Nutrition Info per Serving:
- Calories: 250
- Protein: 5g
- Carbohydrates: 30g
- Fat: 14g
- Fiber: 8g

Servings:
- Serves 4

Cooking Time:
- **Total: 30 minutes**

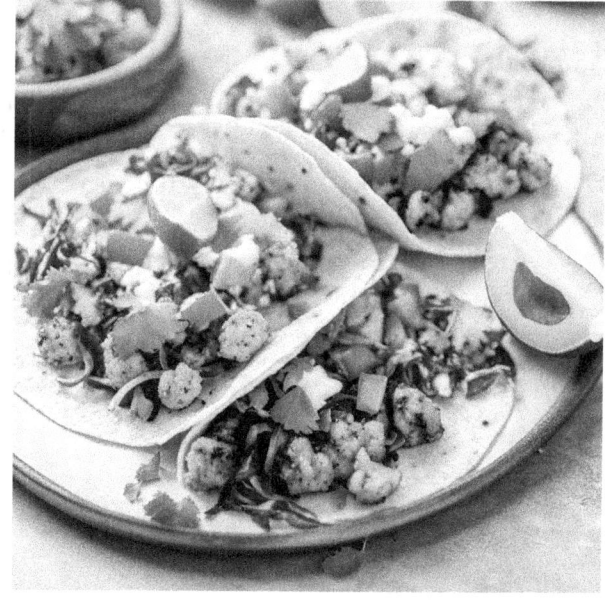

23. Green Bean Almondine

Ingredients:
- 1 pound fresh green beans, trimmed
- 2 tablespoons olive oil
- 2 cloves garlic, minced
- 1/4 cup sliced almonds
- 1 tablespoon lemon juice

Instructions:
1. Bring a large pot of water to a boil. Add the green beans and blanch for 3-4 minutes until tender-crisp. Drain and set aside.
2. In a large skillet, heat the olive oil over medium heat.
3. Add the minced garlic and cook for 1-2 minutes until fragrant.
4. Add the blanched green beans to the skillet and sauté for 3-4 minutes until heated through.
5. Stir in the sliced almonds and cook for another 2 minutes until lightly toasted.
6. Drizzle with lemon juice and toss to combine before serving.

Nutrition Info per Serving:
- Calories: 130
- Protein: 3g
- Carbohydrates: 8g
- Fat: 10g
- Fiber: 4g

Servings:
- Serves 4

Cooking Time:
- Total: 15 minutes

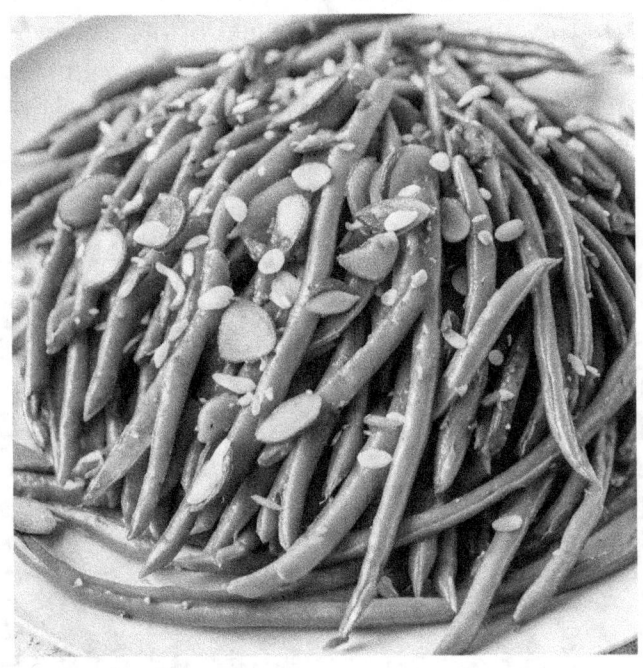

24. Stuffed Portobello Mushrooms with Quinoa

Ingredients:
- 4 large portobello mushrooms, stems removed
- 1 cup cooked quinoa
- 1/2 cup diced tomatoes
- 1/4 cup chopped red onion
- 1/4 cup crumbled feta cheese
- 2 tablespoons olive oil
- 1 teaspoon dried oregano
- 1 tablespoon balsamic vinegar

Instructions:
1. Preheat the oven to 375°F (190°C).
2. In a medium bowl, combine the cooked quinoa, diced tomatoes, chopped red onion, crumbled feta cheese, olive oil, dried oregano, and balsamic vinegar. Mix well.
3. Place the portobello mushrooms on a baking sheet, gill side up.
4. Spoon the quinoa mixture evenly into each mushroom cap.
5. Bake for 20-25 minutes until the mushrooms are tender and the filling is heated through.
6. Serve immediately.

Nutrition Info per Serving:
- Calories: 220
- Protein: 7g
- Carbohydrates: 18g
- Fat: 14g
- Fiber: 4g

Servings:
- Serves 4

Cooking Time:
- Total: 30 minutes

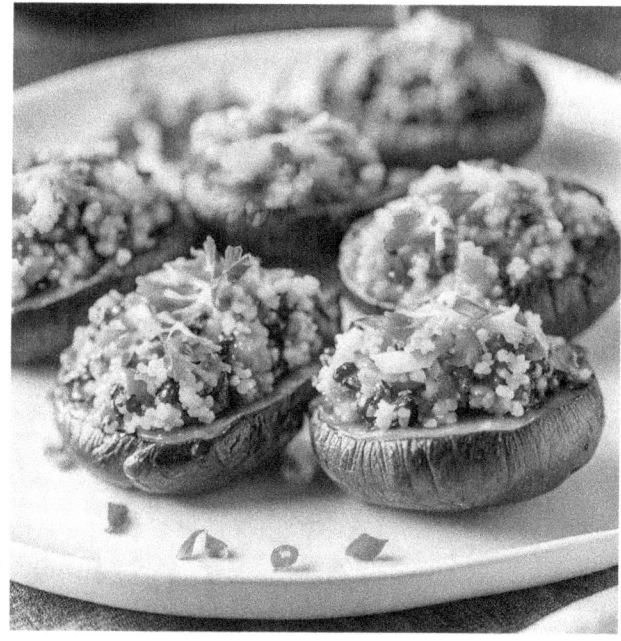

25. Leek and Potato Gratin

Ingredients:
- 2 tablespoons olive oil
- 2 large leeks, white and light green parts only, thinly sliced
- 3 cloves garlic, minced
- 4 large potatoes, thinly sliced
- 1 cup low-fat milk (or dairy-free alternative)
- 1/2 cup grated Parmesan cheese
- 1/4 teaspoon ground nutmeg

Instructions:
1. Preheat the oven to 375°F (190°C).
2. In a large skillet, heat the olive oil over medium heat.
3. Add the sliced leeks and cook until softened, about 5 minutes.
4. Stir in the minced garlic and cook for another 1-2 minutes.
5. In a greased baking dish, layer half of the sliced potatoes.
6. Top with the leek and garlic mixture, then layer the remaining potato slices.
7. In a small bowl, whisk together the milk, grated Parmesan cheese, and ground nutmeg.
8. Pour the milk mixture over the layered potatoes and leeks.
9. Cover the baking dish with foil and bake for 45 minutes.
10. Remove the foil and bake for an additional 15 minutes until the top is golden brown and the potatoes are tender.
11. Allow to cool slightly before serving.

Nutrition Info per Serving:
- Calories: 250
- Protein: 6g
- Carbohydrates: 38g
- Fat: 8g
- Fiber: 4g

Servings:
- Serves 6

Cooking Time:
- Total: 1 hour

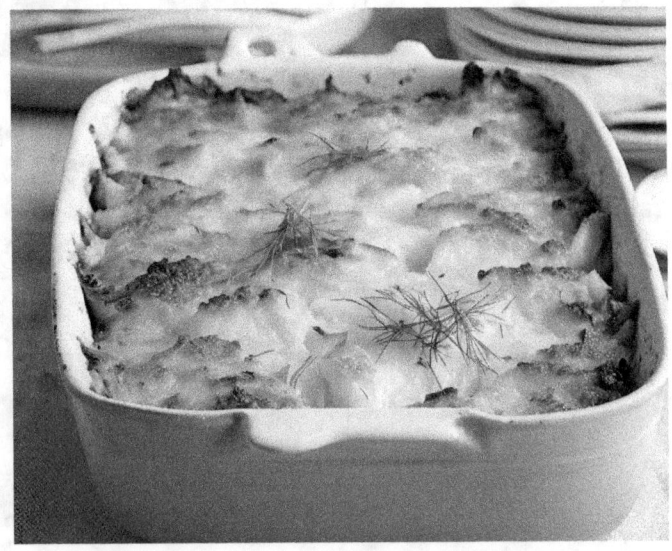

10-WEEK MEAL PLAN

Week 1
Monday
- Breakfast: Greek Yogurt Parfait with Nuts and Berries
- Lunch: Shrimp and Avocado Salad
- Dinner: Balsamic Glazed Chicken Breasts with a side of Roasted Cauliflower with Turmeric and Cumin

Tuesday
- Breakfast: Spinach and Feta Omelette
- Lunch: Turkey Lettuce Wraps
- Dinner: Grilled Salmon with Lemon Dill Sauce with a side of Green Bean Almondine

Wednesday
- Breakfast: Almond Butter Banana Smoothie
- Lunch: Greek Yogurt Parfait with Nuts and Berries
- Dinner: Baked Cod with Herb Crust with a side of Roasted Parsnips and Carrots with Honey Glaze

Thursday
- Breakfast: Turkey and Spinach Scramble
- Lunch: Tomato Gazpacho
- Dinner: Spicy Shrimp Stir-Fry with a side of Stir-Fried Bok Choy with Garlic and Soy Sauce

Friday
- Breakfast: Protein Pancakes
- Lunch: Beetroot and Feta Salad
- Dinner: Pistachio-Crusted Halibut with a side of Cabbage Slaw with Apple Cider Vinegar Dressing

Saturday
- Breakfast: Vegetable Stir-Fry with Tofu
- Lunch: Stuffed Bell Peppers with Brown Rice and Vegetables
- Dinner: Chicken and Spinach Stuffed Sweet Potatoes

Sunday
- Breakfast: Quinoa Porridge
- Lunch: Vegan Cauliflower Tacos
- Dinner: Lemon Garlic Turkey Burgers with a side of Kale and Quinoa Salad with Lemon Vinaigrette

Week 2

Monday
- Breakfast: Egg Muffins with Veggies and Cheese
- Lunch: Tuna Nicoise Salad
- Dinner: Fish Tacos with Cabbage Slaw with a side of Green Bean Almondine

Tuesday
- Breakfast: Kale and Sweet Potato Hash
- Lunch: Turkey Meatball Soup
- Dinner: Chicken Ratatouille with a side of Roasted Cauliflower with Turmeric and Cumin

Wednesday
- Breakfast: Low Carb Blueberry Muffins
- Lunch: Stuffed Portobello Mushrooms with Quinoa
- Dinner: Seafood Paella with a side of Green Bean Almondine

Thursday
- Breakfast: Zucchini and Carrot Fritters
- Lunch: Balsamic Glazed Chicken Breasts
- Dinner: Mushroom and Spinach Stuffed Chicken with a side of Cucumber and Dill Salad with Yogurt Dressing

Friday
- Breakfast: Overnight Oats with Flaxseed
- Lunch: Chicken Sausage Breakfast Burrito
- Dinner: Curried Chicken Salad with a side of Green Bean Almondine

Saturday
- Breakfast: Chicken and Spinach Stuffed Sweet Potatoes
- Lunch: Grilled Shrimp and Pineapple Skewers
- Dinner: Seared Scallops with Mango Salsa with a side of Roasted Parsnips and Carrots with Honey Glaze

Sunday
- Breakfast: Tempeh and Broccoli Saute
- Lunch: Egg Muffins with Veggies and Cheese
- Dinner: Sweet Potato and Chickpea Curry with a side of Stir-Fried Bok Choy with Garlic and Soy Sauce

Week 3

Monday
- Breakfast: Almond Flour Waffles
- Lunch: Chicken and Vegetable Stir-Fry
- Dinner: BBQ Turkey Meatloaf with a side of Green Bean Almondine

Tuesday
- Breakfast: Oat Bran Muffin
- Lunch: Baked Lemon Herb Chicken
- Dinner: Lemon Pepper Haddock with a side of Cabbage Slaw with Apple Cider Vinegar Dressing

Wednesday
- Breakfast: Grilled Mackerel with Orange Salad
- Lunch: Vegetable Paella with Saffron
- Dinner: Sweet Potato and Chickpea Curry with a side of Green Bean Almondine

Thursday
- Breakfast: Spinach and Feta Omelette
- Lunch: Stuffed Bell Peppers with Brown Rice and Vegetables
- Dinner: Chicken Ratatouille with a side of Stir-Fried Bok Choy with Garlic and Soy Sauce

Friday
- Breakfast: Greek Yogurt Parfait with Nuts and Berries
- Lunch: Shrimp and Avocado Salad
- Dinner: Spicy Chicken and Hummus Pita with a side of Green Bean Almondine

Saturday
- Breakfast: Quinoa Porridge
- Lunch: Chicken and Broccoli Alfredo
- Dinner: Lemon Garlic Butter Scallops with a side of Roasted Parsnips and Carrots with Honey Glaze

Sunday
- Breakfast: Low Carb Blueberry Muffins
- Lunch: Fish Tacos with Cabbage Slaw
- Dinner: Thai Coconut Fish Soup with a side of Green Bean Almondine

Week 4

Monday
- Breakfast: Almond Butter Banana Smoothie
- Lunch: Turkey Lettuce Wraps
- Dinner: Cajun Chicken Quinoa Bowl with a side of Green Bean Almondine

Tuesday
- Breakfast: Pumpkin Seed Granola
- Lunch: Tuna Nicoise Salad
- Dinner: Grilled Salmon with Lemon Dill Sauce with a side of Stir-Fried Bok Choy with Garlic and Soy Sauce

Wednesday
- Breakfast: Soy and Linseed Porridge
- Lunch: Baked Cod with Herb Crust
- Dinner: Curried Lentils with Spinach and Carrots with a side of Green Bean Almondine

Thursday
- Breakfast: Buckwheat Pancakes
- Lunch: Turkey Meatball Soup
- Dinner: Grilled Shrimp and Pineapple Skewers with a side of Cabbage Slaw with Apple Cider Vinegar Dressing

Friday
- Breakfast: Beetroot and Ginger Smoothie
- Lunch: Mushroom and Barley Soup
- Dinner: Chicken and Lentil Stew with a side of Green Bean Almondine

Saturday
- Breakfast: Tuna Salad on Whole Wheat Toast
- Lunch: Spinach and Mushroom Quiche
- Dinner: Spicy Shrimp Stir-Fry with a side of Roasted Parsnips and Carrots with Honey Glaze

Sunday
- Breakfast: Kale and Sweet Potato Hash
- Lunch: Grilled Eggplant with Tahini Sauce
- Dinner: Seared Scallops with Mango Salsa with a side of Green Bean Almondine

Week 5

Monday
- Breakfast: Tempeh and Broccoli Saute
- Lunch: Cucumber and Dill Salad with Yogurt Dressing
- Dinner: BBQ Turkey Meatloaf with a side of Green Bean Almondine

Tuesday
- Breakfast: Almond Flour Waffles
- Lunch: Chicken Ratatouille
- Dinner: Pistachio-Crusted Halibut with a side of Stir-Fried Bok Choy with Garlic and Soy Sauce

Wednesday
- Breakfast: Oat Bran Muffin
- Lunch: Fish Tacos with Cabbage Slaw
- Dinner: Sweet Potato and Chickpea Curry with a side of Green Bean Almondine

Thursday
- Breakfast: Grilled Mackerel with Orange Salad
- Lunch: Tuna Nicoise Salad
- Dinner: Chicken and Spinach Stuffed Sweet Potatoes with a side of Cabbage Slaw with Apple Cider Vinegar Dressing

Friday
- Breakfast: Greek Yogurt Parfait with Nuts and Berries
- Lunch: Shrimp and Avocado Salad
- Dinner: Lemon Pepper Haddock with a side of Green Bean Almondine

Saturday
- Breakfast: Zucchini Noodles with Pesto and Cherry Tomatoes
- Lunch: Vegetable Paella with Saffron
- Dinner: Curried Chicken Salad with a side of Green Bean Almondine

Sunday
- Breakfast: Pumpkin Seed Granola
- Lunch: Stuffed Portobello Mushrooms with Quinoa
- Dinner: Spicy Shrimp Stir-Fry with a side of Roasted Parsnips and Carrots with Honey Glaze

Week 6

Monday
- Breakfast: Egg Muffins with Veggies and Cheese
- Lunch: Spinach and Feta Omelette
- Dinner: Turkey and Sweet Potato Skillet with a side of Roasted Cauliflower with Turmeric and Cumin

Tuesday
- Breakfast: Almond Butter Banana Smoothie
- Lunch: Curried Lentils with Spinach and Carrots
- Dinner: Lemon Garlic Butter Scallops with a side of Green Bean Almondine

Wednesday
- Breakfast: Quinoa Porridge
- Lunch: Vegan Cauliflower Tacos
- Dinner: Balsamic Glazed Chicken Breasts with a side of Stir-Fried Bok Choy with Garlic and Soy Sauce

Thursday
- Breakfast: Tempeh and Broccoli Saute
- Lunch: Beetroot and Feta Salad
- Dinner: Chicken and Vegetable Stir-Fry with a side of Roasted Parsnips and Carrots with Honey Glaze

Friday
- Breakfast: Low Carb Blueberry Muffins
- Lunch: Turkey Meatball Soup
- Dinner: Fish Tacos with Cabbage Slaw with a side of Cucumber and Dill Salad with Yogurt Dressing

Saturday
- Breakfast: Spinach and Mushroom Quiche
- Lunch: Chicken and Spinach Stuffed Sweet Potatoes
- Dinner: Grilled Shrimp and Pineapple Skewers with a side of Green Bean Almondine

Sunday
- Breakfast: Zucchini Noodles with Pesto and Cherry Tomatoes
- Lunch: Tuna Nicoise Salad
- Dinner: Mushroom and Barley Soup with a side of Roasted Parsnips and Carrots with Honey Glaze

Week 7
Monday
- Breakfast: Pumpkin Seed Granola
- Lunch: Curried Chicken Salad
- Dinner: Seared Scallops with Mango Salsa with a side of Green Bean Almondine

Tuesday
- Breakfast: Soy and Linseed Porridge
- Lunch: Stuffed Portobello Mushrooms with Quinoa
- Dinner: Thai Coconut Fish Soup with a side of Stir-Fried Bok Choy with Garlic and Soy Sauce

Wednesday
- Breakfast: Buckwheat Pancakes
- Lunch: Chicken Sausage Breakfast Burrito
- Dinner: Spicy Shrimp Stir-Fry with a side of Green Bean Almondine

Thursday
- Breakfast: Beetroot and Ginger Smoothie
- Lunch: Baked Lemon Herb Chicken
- Dinner: BBQ Turkey Meatloaf with a side of Roasted Parsnips and Carrots with Honey Glaze

Friday
- Breakfast: Tuna Salad on Whole Wheat Toast
- Lunch: Grilled Mackerel with Orange Salad
- Dinner: Baked Cod with Herb Crust with a side of Cabbage Slaw with Apple Cider Vinegar Dressing

Saturday
- Breakfast: Kale and Sweet Potato Hash
- Lunch: Seared Scallops with Mango Salsa
- Dinner: Lemon Pepper Haddock with a side of Green Bean Almondine

Sunday
- Breakfast: Almond Flour Waffles
- Lunch: Turkey Lettuce Wraps
- Dinner: Chicken and Lentil Stew with a side of Stir-Fried Bok Choy with Garlic and Soy Sauce

Week 8

Monday
- Breakfast: Pumpkin Seed Granola
- Lunch: Grilled Eggplant with Tahini Sauce
- Dinner: Grilled Salmon with Lemon Dill Sauce with a side of Roasted Parsnips and Carrots with Honey Glaze

Tuesday
- Breakfast: Oat Bran Muffin
- Lunch: Tomato Gazpacho
- Dinner: Lemon Garlic Turkey Burgers with a side of Cabbage Slaw with Apple Cider Vinegar Dressing

Wednesday
- Breakfast: Grilled Mackerel with Orange Salad
- Lunch: Spinach and Mushroom Quiche
- Dinner: Sweet Potato and Chickpea Curry with a side of Green Bean Almondine

Thursday
- Breakfast: Soy and Linseed Porridge
- Lunch: Shrimp and Avocado Salad
- Dinner: Spicy Chicken and Hummus Pita with a side of Stir-Fried Bok Choy with Garlic and Soy Sauce

Friday
- Breakfast: Greek Yogurt Parfait with Nuts and Berries
- Lunch: Vegan Cauliflower Tacos
- Dinner: Baked Lemon Herb Chicken with a side of Cucumber and Dill Salad with Yogurt Dressing

Saturday
- Breakfast: Zucchini Noodles with Pesto and Cherry Tomatoes
- Lunch: Mushroom and Barley Soup
- Dinner: Spicy Shrimp Stir-Fry with a side of Green Bean Almondine

Sunday
- Breakfast: Almond Butter Banana Smoothie
- Lunch: Curried Lentils with Spinach and Carrots
- Dinner: Pistachio-Crusted Halibut with a side of Roasted Parsnips and Carrots with Honey Glaze

Week 9

Monday
- Breakfast: Greek Yogurt Parfait with Nuts and Berries
- Lunch: Spinach and Feta Omelette
- Dinner: Cajun Chicken Quinoa Bowl with a side of Green Bean Almondine

Tuesday
- Breakfast: Low Carb Blueberry Muffins
- Lunch: Curried Chicken Salad
- Dinner: Seared Scallops with Mango Salsa with a side of Cabbage Slaw with Apple Cider Vinegar Dressing

Wednesday
- Breakfast: Quinoa Porridge
- Lunch: Vegan Cauliflower Tacos
- Dinner: Balsamic Glazed Chicken Breasts with a side of Stir-Fried Bok Choy with Garlic and Soy Sauce

Thursday
- Breakfast: Tempeh and Broccoli Saute
- Lunch: Beetroot and Feta Salad
- Dinner: Chicken and Vegetable Stir-Fry with a side of Roasted Parsnips and Carrots with Honey Glaze

Friday
- Breakfast: Pumpkin Seed Granola
- Lunch: Tomato Gazpacho
- Dinner: Lemon Garlic Butter Scallops with a side of Green Bean Almondine

Saturday
- Breakfast: Spinach and Mushroom Quiche
- Lunch: Chicken Sausage Breakfast Burrito
- Dinner: Spicy Shrimp Stir-Fry with a side of Cabbage Slaw with Apple Cider Vinegar Dressing

Sunday
- Breakfast: Kale and Sweet Potato Hash
- Lunch: Tuna Nicoise Salad
- Dinner: Sweet Potato and Chickpea Curry with a side of Green Bean Almondine

Week 10

Monday
- Breakfast: Almond Butter Banana Smoothie
- Lunch: Shrimp and Avocado Salad
- Dinner: Lemon Pepper Haddock with a side of Stir-Fried Bok Choy with Garlic and Soy Sauce

Tuesday
- Breakfast: Tempeh and Broccoli Saute
- Lunch: Beetroot and Feta Salad
- Dinner: Grilled Salmon with Lemon Dill Sauce with a side of Roasted Parsnips and Carrots with Honey Glaze

Wednesday
- Breakfast: Almond Flour Waffles
- Lunch: Spinach and Mushroom Quiche
- Dinner: Seared Scallops with Mango Salsa with a side of Green Bean Almondine

Thursday
- Breakfast: Soy and Linseed Porridge
- Lunch: Turkey Meatball Soup
- Dinner: Chicken and Lentil Stew with a side of Cucumber and Dill Salad with Yogurt Dressing

Friday
- Breakfast: Buckwheat Pancakes
- Lunch: Stuffed Portobello Mushrooms with Quinoa
- Dinner: Baked Lemon Herb Chicken with a side of Stir-Fried Bok Choy with Garlic and Soy Sauce

Saturday
- Breakfast: Greek Yogurt Parfait with Nuts and Berries
- Lunch: Grilled Eggplant with Tahini Sauce
- Dinner: Sweet Potato and Chickpea Curry with a side of Green Bean Almondine

Sunday
- Breakfast: Zucchini Noodles with Pesto and Cherry Tomatoes
- Lunch: Tomato Gazpacho
- Dinner: Pistachio-Crusted Halibut with a side of Roasted Parsnips and Carrots with Honey Glaze

Weekly Meal planner + Journal

	BREAKFAST	LUNCH	DINNER	SNACKS
MON				
TUE				
WED				
THU				
FRI				
SAT				
SUN				

Describe your current daily eating habits. What foods do you commonly consume for breakfast, lunch, and dinner?

....

....

....

....

....

....

....

Weekly Meal planner + Journal

	BREAKFAST	LUNCH	DINNER	SNACKS
MON				
TUE				
WED				
THU				
FRI				
SAT				
SUN				

What are your main goals for starting the narcolepsy diet? How do you hope it will affect your daily life and symptoms?

....
....
....
....
....
....
....

Weekly Meal planner + Journal

	BREAKFAST	LUNCH	DINNER	SNACKS
MON				
TUE				
WED				
THU				
FRI				
SAT				
SUN				

List any foods that you have noticed trigger your narcolepsy symptoms. How do these foods affect you?

....

....

....

....

....

....

....

Weekly Meal planner + Journal

	BREAKFAST	LUNCH	DINNER	SNACKS
MON				
TUE				
WED				
THU				
FRI				
SAT				
SUN				

How often do you experience daytime sleepiness? Do you notice a correlation between your meals and your energy levels?

....
....
....
....
....
....
....

Weekly Meal planner + Journal

	BREAKFAST	LUNCH	DINNER	SNACKS
MON				
TUE				
WED				
THU				
FRI				
SAT				
SUN				

What challenges do you anticipate facing while following the narcolepsy diet? How do you plan to overcome these challenges?

....
....
....
....
....
....
....

Weekly Meal planner + Journal

	BREAKFAST	LUNCH	DINNER	SNACKS
MON				
TUE				
WED				
THU				
FRI				
SAT				
SUN				

Write down a typical grocery list that aligns with the narcolepsy diet. How does this list differ from your usual grocery shopping?

....

....

....

....

....

....

....

Weekly Meal planner + Journal

	BREAKFAST	LUNCH	DINNER	SNACKS
MON				
TUE				
WED				
THU				
FRI				
SAT				
SUN				

How will you ensure you stay hydrated throughout the day? What strategies can you use to remind yourself to drink enough water?

....
....
....
....
....
....
....

Weekly Meal planner + Journal

	BREAKFAST	LUNCH	DINNER	SNACKS
MON				
TUE				
WED				
THU				
FRI				
SAT				
SUN				

Reflect on your eating schedule. Do you think adjusting the timing of your meals could help manage your narcolepsy symptoms? Why or why not?

....

....

....

....

....

....

....

Weekly Meal planner + Journal

	BREAKFAST	LUNCH	DINNER	SNACKS
MON				
TUE				
WED				
THU				
FRI				
SAT				
SUN				

Describe a challenging social situation where you might struggle to stick to the narcolepsy diet (e.g., dining out, parties). How will you handle this situation?

....

....

....

....

....

....

....

After a week on the narcolepsy diet, reflect on any changes in your symptoms and energy levels. What positive changes have you noticed, and what adjustments do you still need to make?

Scan the QR code below to get a surprise bonus